CONSIDERATIONS FOR VIRAL DISEASE ERADICATION

Lessons Learned and Future Strategies

Workshop Summary

Stacey Knobler, Joshua Lederberg, and Leslie A. Pray, *Editors*

Forum on Emerging Infections

Board on Global Health

INSTITUTE OF MEDICINE

NATIONAL ACADEMY PRESS
Washington, D.C.

NATIONAL ACADEMY PRESS 2101 Constitution Avenue, N.W. Washington, DC 20418

NOTICE: The project that is the subject of this report was approved by the Governing Board of the National Research Council, whose members are drawn from the councils of the National Academy of Sciences, the National Academy of Engineering, and the Institute of Medicine.

Support for this project was provided by the U.S. Department of Health and Human Services' National Institutes of Health, Centers for Disease Control and Prevention, and Food and Drug Administration; U.S. Department of Defense; U.S. Department of State; U.S. Department of Veterans Affairs; U.S. Agency for International Development; Abbott Laboratories; American Society for Microbiology; Bristol-Myers Squibb Company; Burroughs Wellcome Fund, Eli Lilly & Company; The Ellison Medical Foundation; Glaxo Wellcome; F. Hoffmann-La Roche AG; Pfizer, Inc.; SmithKline Beecham Corporation; and Wyeth-Ayerst Laboratories. The views presented in this report are those of the Institute of Medicine Forum on Emerging Infections and are not necessarily those of the funding agencies.

This report is based on the proceedings of a workshop that was sponsored by the Forum on Emerging Infections. It is prepared in the form of a workshop summary by and in the name of the editors, with the assistance of staff and consultants, as an individually authored document. Sections of the workshop summary not specifically attributed to an individual reflect the views of the editors and not those of the Forum on Emerging Infections. The content of those sections is based on the presentations and the discussions that took place during the workshop.

Library of Congress Cataloging-in-Publication Data

Considerations for viral disease eradication : lessons learned and future strategies : workshop summary / Stacey Knobler, Joshua Lederberg, and Leslie A. Pray, editors ; Forum on Emerging Infections, Board on Global Health, Institute of Medicine.
p. ; cm.
Includes bibliographical references.
ISBN 0-309-08414-8 (pbk.)
1. Virus diseases—Vaccination—Congresses. 2. Virus diseases—Prevention—Congresses. 3. Medical policy—Congresses.
[DNLM: 1. Communicable Disease Control—trends—Congresses. 2. Immunization—trends—Congresses. 3. Virus Diseases—prevention & control—Congresses. 4. Health Policy—Congresses. 5. World Health—Congresses. WA 110 C755 2002] I. Knobler, Stacey. II. Lederberg, Joshua. III. Pray, Leslie A. IV. Institute of Medicine (U.S.). Forum on Emerging Infections.
RA644.V55 C66 2002
614.5'75—dc21

2002005549

Additional copies of this report are available for sale from the National Academy Press, 2101 Constitution Avenue, N.W., Box 285, Washington, DC 20055. Call (800) 624-6242 or (202) 334-3313 (in the Washington metropolitan area), or visit the NAP's home page at **www.nap.edu.** The full text of this report is available at **www.nap.edu.**

For more information about the Institute of Medicine, visit the IOM home page at **www.iom.edu.**

Printed in the United States of America

The serpent has been a symbol of long life, healing, and knowledge among almost all cultures and religions since the beginning of recorded history. The serpent adopted as a logotype by the Institute of Medicine is a relief carving from ancient Greece, now held by the Staatliche Museen in Berlin.

COVER: The background for the cover of this workshop summary is a photograph of a batik designed and printed specifically for the Malaysian Society of Parasitology and Tropical Medicine. The print contains drawings of various parasites and insects; it is used with the kind permission of the Society.

"Knowing is not enough; we must apply.
Willing is not enough; we must do."
—Goethe

INSTITUTE OF MEDICINE

Shaping the Future for Health

THE NATIONAL ACADEMIES

National Academy of Sciences
National Academy of Engineering
Institute of Medicine
National Research Council

The **National Academy of Sciences** is a private, nonprofit, self-perpetuating society of distinguished scholars engaged in scientific and engineering research, dedicated to the furtherance of science and technology and to their use for the general welfare. Upon the authority of the charter granted to it by the Congress in 1863, the Academy has a mandate that requires it to advise the federal government on scientific and technical matters. Dr. Bruce M. Alberts is president of the National Academy of Sciences.

The **National Academy of Engineering** was established in 1964, under the charter of the National Academy of Sciences, as a parallel organization of outstanding engineers. It is autonomous in its administration and in the selection of its members, sharing with the National Academy of Sciences the responsibility for advising the federal government. The National Academy of Engineering also sponsors engineering programs aimed at meeting national needs, encourages education and research, and recognizes the superior achievements of engineers. Dr. Wm. A. Wulf is president of the National Academy of Engineering.

The **Institute of Medicine** was established in 1970 by the National Academy of Sciences to secure the services of eminent members of appropriate professions in the examination of policy matters pertaining to the health of the public. The Institute acts under the responsibility given to the National Academy of Sciences by its congressional charter to be an adviser to the federal government and, upon its own initiative, to identify issues of medical care, research, and education. Dr. Harvey V. Fineberg is president of the Institute of Medicine.

The **National Research Council** was organized by the National Academy of Sciences in 1916 to associate the broad community of science and technology with the Academy's purposes of furthering knowledge and advising the federal government. Functioning in accordance with general policies determined by the Academy, the Council has become the principal operating agency of both the National Academy of Sciences and the National Academy of Engineering in providing services to the government, the public, and the scientific and engineering communities. The Council is administered jointly by both Academies and the Institute of Medicine. Dr. Bruce M. Alberts and Dr. Wm. A. Wulf are chairman and vice chairman, respectively, of the National Research Council.

FORUM ON EMERGING INFECTIONS

LYNN MARKS, Global Head of Infectious Diseases, GlaxoSmithKline, Collegeville, Pennsylvania
STEPHEN MORSE, Director, Center for Public Health Preparedness, Columbia University, New York, New York
MICHAEL OSTERHOLM, Director, Center for Infectious Disease Research and Policy and Professor, School of Public Health, University of Minnesota, Minneapolis, Minnesota
GARY ROSELLE, Program Director for Infectious Diseases, VA Central Office, Veterans Health Administration, Department of Veterans Affairs, Washington, D.C.
DAVID SHLAES, Vice President, Infectious Disease Research, Wyeth, Pearl River, New York
JANET SHOEMAKER, Director, Office of Public Affairs, American Society for Microbiology, Washington, D.C.
P. FREDRICK SPARLING, J. Herbert Bate Professor Emeritus of Medicine, Microbiology, and Immunology, University of North Carolina, Chapel Hill, North Carolina
KAYE WACHSMUTH, Deputy Administrator, Office of Public Health and Science, United States Department of Agriculture, Washington, D.C.
C. DOUGLAS WEBB, Senior Medical Director, Bristol-Myers Squibb Company, Princeton, New Jersey

Liaisons to the Forum

ENRIQUETA BOND, President, Burroughs Wellcome Fund, Research Triangle Park, North Carolina
NANCY CARTER-FOSTER, Director, Program for Emerging Infections and HIV/AIDS, U.S. Department of State, Washington, D.C.
MICHAEL HORAN, Associate Vice President of Clinical Affairs, Pharmaceutical Research and Manufacturers Association, Washington, D.C.
EDWARD McSWEEGAN, National Institute of Allergy and Infectious Diseases, National Institutes of Health, Bethesda, Maryland
STEPHEN OSTROFF, Associate Director for Epidemiologic Science, National Center for Infectious Diseases, Centers for Disease Control and Prevention, Atlanta, Georgia
FRED TENOVER, Chief, Nosocomial Pathogens Laboratory Branch, National Center for Infectious Diseases, Centers for Disease Control and Prevention, Atlanta, Georgia

Staff

JONATHAN DAVIS, Senior Program Officer (until May 2001)
STACEY KNOBLER, Director, Forum on Emerging Infections
MARJAN NAJAFI, Research Associate
LAURIE SPINELLI, Project Assistant

Reviewers

This report has been reviewed in draft form by individuals chosen for their diverse perspectives and technical expertise, in accordance with procedures approved by the National Research Council's Report Review Committee. The purpose of this independent review is to provide candid and critical comments that will assist the institution in making its published report as sound as possible and to ensure that the report meets institutional standards for objectivity, evidence, and responsiveness to the study charge. The review comments and draft manuscript remain confidential to protect the integrity of the deliberative process. We wish to thank the following individuals for their review of this report:

Jon Andrus, University of California, San Francisco, CA
Kenneth Bernard, Office of Senator Frist, U.S. Senate, Washington, D.C.
David Heymann, World Health Organization, Geneva, Switzerland
Walter Orenstein, Centers for Disease Control and Prevention, Atlanta, GA
Murray Trostle, U.S. Agency for International Development, Washington, D.C.

Although the reviewers listed above have provided many constructive comments and suggestions, they were not asked to endorse the final draft of the report before its release. The review of this report was overseen by Charles Carpenter, M.D. Appointed by the National Research Council, he was responsible for making certain that an independent examination of this report was carried out in accordance with institutional procedures and that all review comments were carefully considered. Responsibility for the final content of this report rests entirely with the authoring committee and the institution.

Contents

APPENDIXES

Preface

The Forum on Emerging Infections was created in 1996 in response to a request from the Centers for Disease Control and Prevention and the National Institutes of Health. The goal of the Forum is to provide structured opportunities for representatives from academia, industry, professional and interest groups, and government[1] to examine and discuss scientific and policy issues that are of shared interest and that are specifically related to research and prevention, detection, and management of emerging infectious diseases. In accomplishing this task, the Forum provides the opportunity to foster the exchange of information and ideas, identify areas in need of greater attention, clarify policy issues by enhancing knowledge and identifying points of agreement, and inform decision makers about science and policy issues. The Forum seeks to illuminate issues rather than resolve them directly; hence, it does not provide advice or recommendations on any specific policy initiative pending before any agency or organization. Its strengths are the diversity of its membership and the contributions of individual members expressed throughout the activities of the Forum.

[1]Representatives of federal agencies serve in an *ex officio* capacity. An *ex officio* member of a group is one who is a member automatically by virtue of holding a particular office or membership in another body.

ABOUT THE WORKSHOP

The legacy of smallpox eradication has removed the worldwide suffering caused by this disease, has resulted in yearly savings of substantial financial resources that are no longer needed for its treatment and prevention, and has helped build consensus and confidence to expand eradication programs to other diseases. Since smallpox eradication, the science of eradication has changed and with it, our definitions of what diseases are possible to eradicate. For example, many diseases, such as polio, measles, onchocerciasis, dracunculiasis, lymphatic filariasis, leprosy, and Chagas diseases, once thought not to be eradicable, are now targeted for elimination and subsequent eradication.[2] These and other disease control experiences provide strong evidence that with full implementation of an appropriate control strategy, disease transmission can be effectively interrupted, if not eliminated regionally and possibly eradicated globally.

Among the vaccine-preventable diseases, concerted efforts are underway to eliminate or eradicate several viral diseases. By 2002, it is anticipated that wild type poliovirus transmission will be interrupted worldwide. The Pan American Health Organization (PAHO) in 1994 developed an enhanced measles vaccination strategy with the goal of measles elimination from the Western Hemisphere by 2000. While measles cases are still reported, PAHO's measles elimination strategy has been very effective in interrupting transmission and maintaining the absence of measles virus in >99% of the 12,000 reporting municipalities in the Americas. The interruption of indigenous measles transmission in the Americas by the end of the year 2001 remains an attainable goal.

The criteria for assessing eradicability of polio, measles, and other viral infections have been debated extensively. What is specifically not addressed are the relative desirability and feasibility, and the time required, for stopping immunizations. With the elimination and eradication of several viral diseases on the horizon, issues surrounding the cessation of immunization activities become exceedingly important. Resolution of the issues affecting when and how immunization and other prevention activities can be stopped in conjunction with disease eradication are paramount to domestic and

---

[2]In 1997, the Dahlem Workshop on the Eradication of Infectious Diseases defined several levels of deliberate efforts of disease control, including eradication, as follows: *Control*: reduction of disease incidence, prevalence, morbidity, and mortality to acceptable levels; *Elimination of disease*: reduction to zero incidence of disease in a defined geographic area; *Elimination of infection*: reduction to zero incidence of infection caused by a specific agent in a defined geographic area; *Eradication*: permanent reduction to zero worldwide incidence of infection caused by a specific agent; *Extinction*: the specific agent no longer exists in nature or the laboratory. It is important to note that within the following authored papers there is some inconsistency among the interpretations of these definitions.

international public health agencies, pharmaceutical and vaccine manufacturers, and security analysts.

In an effort to better understand the dynamics of disease eradication and post-immunization policies, the Institute of Medicine (IOM)'s Forum on Emerging Infections hosted a two-day workshop (February 1–2, 2001) on *The Consequences of Viral Disease Eradication*. Through invited presentations, panel discussion, and open dialogue with workshop participants, we explored the principles underlying the biological challenges, medical interventions, and operational considerations for post-immunization strategies for vaccine-preventable viral diseases, and highlighted important efforts that may facilitate wise decision making.

ORGANIZATION OF WORKSHOP SUMMARY

This workshop summary report is prepared for the Forum membership in the name of the editors, with the assistance of staff and consultants, as an individually authored document. Sections of the workshop summary not specifically attributed to an individual reflect the views of the editors and not those of the Forum on Emerging Infections sponsors, or the Institute of Medicine. The contents of the unattributed sections are based on the presentations and discussions that took place during the workshop.

The workshop summary is organized within chapters as a topic-by-topic description of the presentations and discussions. Its purpose is to present lessons from relevant experience, delineate a range of pivotal issues and their respective problems, and put forth some potential responses as described by the workshop participants. The Summary and Assessment chapter discusses the core messages that emerged from the speakers' presentations and the ensuing discussions. Chapter 1 is an introduction and overview of past disease eradication efforts and prospects for the future. Chapters 2 to 6 begin with overviews provided by the editors, followed by the edited presentations made by the invited speakers. Appendix A is a glossary and list of acronyms useful to the reader. Appendix B presents the workshop agenda. Forum member and speaker biographies are presented in Appendix C.

Although this workshop summary provides an account of the individual presentations, it also reflects an important aspect of the Forum philosophy. The workshop functions as a dialogue among representatives from different sectors and presents their beliefs on which areas may merit further attention. However, the reader should be aware that the material presented here expresses the views and opinions of those participating in the workshop and not the deliberations of a formally constituted IOM study committee. These proceedings summarize only what participants stated in the workshop and are not intended to be an exhaustive exploration of the subject matter.

ACKNOWLEDGMENTS

The Forum on Emerging Infections and the IOM wish to express their warmest appreciation to the individuals and organizations who gave valuable time to provide information and advice to the Forum through participation in the workshop.

The Forum is indebted to the IOM staff who contributed during the course of the workshop and the production of this workshop summary. On behalf of the Forum, I gratefully acknowledge the efforts led by Stacey Knobler and Jonathan Davis, who dedicated much effort and time to developing this workshop's agenda and for their thoughtful and insightful approach and skill in translating the workshop proceedings and discussion into this workshop summary. I would also like to thank the following IOM staff and consultants for their valuable contributions to this activity: Leslie Pray, Marjan Najafi, Laurie Spinelli, Judith Bale, Katherine Oberholtzer, Paige Baldwin, Jennifer Otten, Brett Marvin, Clyde Behney, Bronwyn Schrecker, Sally Stanfield, Francesca Moghari, Estelle Miller, and Beth Gyorgy.

Finally, the Forum also thanks sponsors that supported this activity. Financial support for this project was provided by the U.S. Department of Health and Human Services' National Institutes of Health, Centers for Disease Control and Prevention, and the Food and Drug Administration; U.S. Department of Defense; U.S. Department of State; U.S. Agency for International Development; U.S. Department of Veterans Affairs; Abbott Laboratories; American Society for Microbiology; Bristol-Myers Squibb Company; Burroughs Wellcome Fund; Eli Lilly & Company; The Ellison Medical Foundation; Glaxo Wellcome; F. Hoffmann-La Roche AG; Pfizer; SmithKline Beecham Corporation; and Wyeth-Ayerst Laboratories. The views presented in this workshop summary are those of the editors and workshop participants and are not necessarily those of the funding organizations.

Joshua Lederberg, Chair
Forum on Emerging Infections

Summary and Assessment

Joshua Lederberg, Ph.D.

Nobel Laureate and Sackler Foundation Scholar
The Rockefeller University, New York, NY

The successful smallpox campaign demonstrates that global eradication of a disease is possible, given the necessary technical base, political commitment, and economic resources for immunization and continued surveillance. Currently, there are three infectious viral disease candidates for global eradication—polio, measles, and rubella—each of which closely satisfies necessary preconditions for eradication as outlined by the 1997 Dahlem Conference on Disease Eradication:

(1) no animal reservoir for the virus is known or suspected;
(2) sensitive and specific tools are available for diagnosis and surveillance;
(3) transmission from one individual to another can be interrupted;
(4) non-lethal infection or vaccination confers life-long immunity;
(5) the burden of disease is important to international public health; and
(6) political commitment to eradication efforts exists.

Of the three diseases, poliomyelitis is likely the next candidate for global eradication. In the Americas, polio was eradicated in the early 1990s, and less than 3,000 cases were reported worldwide in 2000. The current goal is certification of global eradication by 2005. Measles stands next in line after polio, although no global goal has been set. In 2000, there were only 1,500 reported cases of measles in the Americas; however, measles still causes 900,000 deaths each year worldwide and accounts for some 30% of all deaths due to vaccine-preventable diseases. Rubella, which generates 100,000 cases of congenital rubella syndrome, is the furthest from global eradication.

Many attributes of the disease uniquely favored smallpox eradication. Its characteristic clinical features made diagnosis and surveillance for infection much easier than they are for polio, measles, and particularly rubella. Every infected person had a characteristic rash; thus, the presence of the virus in a geographic area could be readily determined. Containment was easy since transmission was by droplets spread by face-to-face contact, and the virus survived outside the human host for only a limited period of time (in contrast to poliovirus, for example, which spreads through a fecal-oral route and may remain viable in feces for six weeks or longer). Smallpox had a higher average age at infection prior to wide-scale vaccination and thus was less transmissible than either polio or measles. A safe, heat-stable vaccine assured protection with only a single inoculation and could be administered from the time of birth (in contrast to oral polio vaccine [OPV], for example, which requires a three-dose regimen and special storage requirements). Finally, an extraordinary international cooperative effort supported the campaign.

Despite these ideal criteria for disease eradication, the smallpox campaign was not without technical, financial, and political challenges. Expected voluntary contributions to the program were sparse in fulfillment. A number of endemic countries needed persuasion to undertake vaccination and surveillance activities, and political and social upheaval seriously delayed or threatened the campaign. It was difficult to achieve sustained interest and support for continued disease surveillance and immunization after a nil incidence was achieved locally, even in light of rumors of sporadic cases and the threat of possible reintroduction. These challenges show that eradication can be extremely difficult even when eradication is technically and operationally feasible and political commitment is strong.

The success of the smallpox eradication campaign and the title of this meeting hint at future success. Indeed, the regional eradication and near-eradication, respectively, of polio and measles in the Americas illustrate tremendous progress. However, it is far from clear that success is just around the corner. Interruption of the final chains of transmission faces several difficult challenges, including high transmissibility in densely populated areas and public and professional complacency regarding continued vaccination due to dwindling first-hand experience with the consequences of infection and the increasing publicity on adverse reactions to vaccination. Even in developed countries where infections have been eradicated or near-eradicated, mass vaccination will probably have to be maintained at very high levels for an extended time in order to protect against reintroduction from areas where poverty, civil unrest, or lack of political will impede high vaccination coverage and sustain endemicity.

There is much concern that the sixth precondition for eradication as outlined at Dahlem—political commitment—is not being fully met with respect to measles and rubella. This is evident by recent discussions among members of the international public health community which reflect serious reservations about the feasibility and cost of attempting to eradicate these two diseases. Indeed, operational feasibility, particularly with regards to maintaining a strong routine immunization program, is considered by many to be an important additional criterion that was omitted from the Dahlem list of preconditions for eradication. As was learned from the Dominican Republic/Haiti polio outbreak, low routine coverage is a critical problem that can lead to the circulation of a virus for several years. Yet, in the case of measles, in many countries the feasibility of delivering routine immunizations is too often ignored by those who advocate eradication. Thus, it is important to note that the current World Health Organization (WHO) strategy for measles is "mortality reduction" and not "eradication". The failure to address the operational aspects of routine coverage seriously threatens our ability to achieve mortality reduction and certainly eradication.

As the title of this report suggests, the focus of this workshop was *post-eradication* challenges. However, certification of eradication for other infectious diseases besides smallpox may be years off. Eradication efforts against polio, measles, and rubella represent a broad spectrum of achievement. The current status of and particular challenges to each were also discussed during the workshop, the highlights of which are presented below.

POLIO

The main challenges confronting global eradication of polio are maintaining high levels of immunization in the population at large (the global polio eradication initiative relies on national immunization days (NIDs) with OPV offered two or more times annually for all children under five years of age) and targeting high-risk areas with "mopping up" operations in order to interrupt the last chains of transmission.

A major lesson from the regional polio eradication effort in the Americas is the need for ongoing analysis of information gathered from the field and for the flexibility to change eradication strategies as necessary. For example, based on information gathered during the campaign, surveillance units were increased and moved to match where patients were seeking initial care. As another example, when it was discovered that a poliovirus type 3 outbreak in Brazil could not be contained by the available vaccine, the manufacturers were led to reformulate the vaccine.

However, as fewer cases are reported, intensified surveillance efforts and immunization programs compete for limited resources with other public health programs, even though laboratory surveillance is critical to the success of the polio global eradication effort. Infection with enteroviruses, echoviruses, and coxsackieviruses can cause an illness whose clinical features emulate paralytic polio, and the OPV vaccine itself can (rarely) cause paralysis. Differentiating OPV-derived viruses and these other causes of paralysis from the wild-type polio virus requires a relatively specialized laboratory technology not readily available in many lesser developed countries. These difficulties confound true incidence rates, encumber surveillance efforts, and consume valuable resources.

Although intensified mopping-up and surveillance have proven to be successful means of interrupting the last chains of polio transmission in the Americas, they were introduced very late in the global program and their implementation elsewhere has been slow. How well we address the challenges of continuing surveillance for poliovirus and in maintaining polio vaccination in polio-free areas until global eradication is achieved will determine whether the goal of certifying the world as polio-free by the year 2005 will be met.

MEASLES

Mathematical models predict that 95% population immunity is needed to interrupt transmission of the measles virus. This is best achieved through a two-dose immunization strategy: once at nine months of age and then again in the second year of life. Major success in prolonged interruption of measles transmission in the Americas using this two-dose immunization strategy, supplemented with nationwide "catch-up" and "follow-up" campaigns targeting susceptible populations and geographic reservoirs, provides evidence for the feasibility of global eradication.

However, several impediments to global measles eradication remain. First, large birth cohorts stay seronegative to measles, resulting in subsequent transmission among a susceptible adult population. Second, virus transmissibility is high in densely populated urban areas where susceptible children and immigrants serve as a source of outbreaks. Third, HIV-infected persons could become chronic carriers of the measles virus and continue to shed the virus long after initial infection. Fourth, more than a million travellers use the skies every day, making it very difficult to contain spread. Fifth, the currently available vaccine is not 100% protective and leaves a pocket of susceptibility that enables transmission.

To address these concerns, research is being done on aerosolization administration and a mucosal route of immunization (versus by injection); however, there is concern about whether the pharmaceutical industry would invest funds in a new vaccine that would entail new manufacturing plants and regulatory compliance and introduction into an unknown market. Also, even if an improved vaccine were developed, the focus of prevention efforts should still be comprehensive immunization of all children.

Sixth, the greatest obstacle to measles eradication may be lack of political will. Indeed, data from the Americas show that measles transmission can be interrupted on entire continents, which means that interruption is technically possible, given the necessary political commitment. While the United States has made measles eradication a public health priority, some of the lowest measles vaccine coverage rates are found among the world's richest countries, where measles is not seen as a problem. These countries need to be encouraged to maintain continued immunization and surveillance as protection against reintroduction via immigration and transcontinental travel. This may require legal mandates. It may also be helpful to compile known risks of vaccination versus disease in some format that is accessible to the public in an effort to assuage concerns about the risks of vaccination. Equally important, health authorities in the developing world need to be confident that embarking on measles eradication will not detract from delivery of other health services and will lead to benefits for overall health care.

As with polio, an important lesson learned from the measles eradication campaign in the Americas is the importance of learning by doing and adjusting strategies based on newly acquired knowledge. For example, measles epidemiology changed radically when immunization was introduced; in particular, its relative incidence increased in older children and young adults. This was particularly true in countries like the United States, where older populations accounted for a greater percentage of cases because of continued susceptibility due either to a lack of vaccination or vaccine failure, coupled with decreased exposure to the wild virus as infants and young children. In response, mass "follow-up" campaigns targeting all children between one and fourteen years of age were recommended every four years in order to remove remaining susceptibility in this older age group and achieve complete interruption of measles transmission.

CONGENITAL RUBELLA SYNDROME

Congenital rubella syndrome (CRS) is a serious disease caused by infection of the fetus with the rubella virus during early pregnancy. Although CRS mortality is not as high as that of measles, the large number of CRS cases (approximately 100,000 worldwide) results in a large population of disabled individuals.

In developed countries, the current strategy of immunization is universal measles-mumps-rubella (MMR) immunization at twelve to eighteen months of age and again at four to twelve years. This strategy has proven successful and should continue. The Pan American Health Organization (PAHO) has recommended that developing countries add rubella to the measles vaccine; increase universal immunization of children between nine and twelve years of age with the combination measles-rubella (MR) vaccine; and repeat mass vaccinations directed at children nine to fourteen years of age. Vaccine manufacturers need to be provided incentives to both decrease the per dose cost and increase the overall supply to meet the demands of increased immunization.

One of the most important challenges to rubella eradication is that clinical diagnosis of rubella is often inaccurate, unlike measles, since rubella can occur without a rash or be completely subclinical. The most sensitive laboratory tools currently available for diagnosis and surveillance are either not suitable for use in the field, can only be used in the most sophisticated laboratories, or are not commercially available. Improved diagnostic capabilities must be developed to accompany rubella eradication.

Another major impediment to CRS eradication is that failure to achieve high immunization coverage in children could lead to increased susceptibility among adult women who have grown up without contact with the virus and thus are more susceptible to infection, which they can then pass on to their fetuses during pregnancy. Ironically, this could potentially lead to more cases of CRS than occurred prior to the implementation of a vaccination program and suggests that it would be prudent to decrease susceptibility in adult women. But this poses a difficult challenge since adult women have an increased risk of reactogenicity and contraindication for use (e.g., possible transmission of live virus to the fetus from vaccination during pregnancy). Experimental work with vector genes and DNA vaccines suggests that maternal immunity could be overcome with the appropriate vaccine. However, there is currently no financial incentive for the pharmaceutical industry to develop a new vaccine or even a new route of administration.

As with measles, garnering broad financial and political support is perhaps the greatest challenge to CRS eradication. Although many years have passed since Australian epidemiologists confirmed CRS, the disabling consequences of CRS are not well publicized, and policymakers in developed countries—where eradication priorities tend to be set—are not as aware of CRS as they are of, for example, polio and measles.

POST-ERADICATION CHALLENGES

Eradication must not beget complacency, but it almost certainly will.

As has been learned from past control or eradication attempts with a variety of viral diseases, from yellow fever to influenza, accidental or intentional reintroduction is a real threat—one that could strike anywhere and for which we need to be fully prepared. This is especially true as immunity wanes in the post-eradication era and the population at large grows more susceptible to infection. Even after immunization ceases, it is crucial that enough vaccine be stockpiled (or provision made for emergency replenishment) to cope with potential outbreaks; that surveillance continues in order to identify and stamp out local outbreaks quickly and before they spread to other regions; that vaccine manufacture be continuously improved to keep up with changing regulatory requirements and new technology; that vital research on vaccine technology and viral biology continue; and that viruses certified as eradicated in the wild be safely contained to minimize the risk of either accidental or intentional reintroduction. Post-eradication strategies need to be carefully developed and implemented in order to secure the full health, human welfare, and economic benefits of the eradication of a viral disease.

Discontinuing immunization in the post-eradication era can yield large cost savings, freeing health care resources for other interventions. However, knowing if, how, and when to stop immunization in the post-eradication era is a major challenge, especially for the polio eradication campaign. Although the use of OPV has been crucial to the success of the polio eradication effort thus far, unique properties of the vaccine complicate decisions regarding if and when to cease vaccination. OPV-derived viruses can revert to pathogenicity during replication in the gut and, if shed, can circulate through the population. The problem of OPV persistence is further complicated by the fact that immunocompromised individuals who are vaccinated with OPV can excrete the virus for unknown, extended lengths of time. Although there is a non-pathogenic alternative to OPV—the inactivated IPV—several practical advantages to OPV make it the vaccine for choice for polio prevention. OPV confers substantial immunity; because it is transmissible, OPV can spread immunity, not just disease; and OPV is much less expensive.

Ideally, a new, non-infectious vaccine that produces mucosal immunity like OPV would be developed as an end-strategy for immunization against polio—perhaps a DNA or some other vectored vaccine—although it is unrealistic to expect either the private or public sector to invest in the development and production of such a vaccine this close to eradication. Different ways of combining OPV and IPV strategies have been considered for use in the post-eradication era, but no decision has been reached about which strategy would offer the best protection against OPV-derived viral disease. For example, one suggested strategy is using an OPV-IPV combination vaccine initially and then eventually removing OPV so that only a "protective IPV layer" remains. However, it is not at all clear that this strategy would ever stop OPV transmission, thus raising the question, should we continue with the cheaper OPV vaccine indefinitely?

Even if IPV could stop OPV transmission, a major disadvantage to relying on IPV as an end-strategy is the enormous cost, considerable technology transfer, and several years that would be required to prepare an adequate supply of IPV to meet the world's needs. With regards to the greater cost of IPV in comparison to OPV, it could be argued that as more new vaccines are introduced into the developing world, the added cost of adding an IPV component may become trivial. One argument for relying on IPV as an end-strategy is that because IPV still allows some intestinal excretion of the poliovirus, the excretion of wild-type virus could be detected in situations where it was believed to have been eradicated. This would facilitate surveillance and detection of outbreaks.

The time is ripe for a decision about how to proceed with vaccine production in the post-eradication era. Will there be an end game, or are we going to vaccinate against polio for the indefinite future? Key to answering this question is knowing whether IPV stops transmission of OPV-derived viruses. It will be ironic if it becomes necessary to continue vaccination in the post-eradication era as protection, not against wild polio, but against polio vaccine-derived disease.

The post-eradication era is one for which we have no historical precedent. We have no experience with the consequences of a reintroduction or reemergence of previously eradicated organisms. We do not know how viruses will evolve in the future; if and how current vaccines would be able to protect us from disease caused by newly evolved viral variants; and if and how our immune system may change as the selective pressures previously imposed by eradicated viruses are lifted or altered. We have no experience on which to base predictions about the rate or extent of spread of disease in a population with zero immunity, especially as increased transcontinental travel and movement of people across borders make containment increasingly difficult. For the first time in human history we have a herd that, for more than twenty years, has never been exposed to epitopes that could potentially reappear in circulation. We need a better understanding of the long-term biological implications of altering the host-virus interaction through eradication and cessation of immunization in the post-eradication era.

Post-eradication strategies need to be developed well before certification of eradication. During the smallpox campaign, post-eradication strategies were developed only after it became clear that the applied vaccine technology had proven successful and that eradication was practical and attainable. That all available resources were devoted towards the goal of interrupting smallpox transmission reflected the strong belief that any strategies that diverted resources away from achieving full eradication would be pointless if the eradication campaign failed. At risk was the loss of billions of dollars invested and gradual reversion to a pre-eradication status as special funds and interest withered. More importantly, a failed eradication effort would have undermined other global initiatives and confidence in expert public health advice. We tend to worry more about the inability to consummate eradication than the consequences of having done so. However, as we have learned, focusing too much on the immediate goal of interrupting transmission without considering the consequences of having done so can leave the population very vulnerable to future public health crises of unpredictable, potentially catastrophic, magnitude.

It has been over 20 years since the global eradication of smallpox. However, several post-eradication challenges remain, including: safely containing virus stocks still being stored in laboratories; renewing abandoned smallpox surveillance efforts; producing a potent vaccine should an outbreak occur; and developing antiviral chemotherapy that might be applicable to smallpox. The risk of reintroduction—especially via biowarfare or bioterrorism—highlights the threat of reversion to a pre-eradication status and the need for developing post-eradication strategies early on during an eradication campaign in order to avoid the need for costly catch-up efforts.

Following eradication, the consequences of reintroduction become increasingly grave over time due to the decline of herd immunity and increased susceptibility of the population to a pandemic, complacency in surveillance and maintenance and improvement of diagnostic laboratories, reduced medical awareness, and decreased research activity.

REINTRODUCTION OF DISEASE IN THE POST-ERADICATION ERA

Reintroduction could strike anywhere, at any time. Bioterrorism is generally considered the greatest risk of smallpox reintroduction, even though it was initially dismissed as a possibility since all countries had actively participated in eradication efforts. By the mid-1990s, however, U.S. intelligence had learned of several countries that were considering using smallpox as a potential bioweapons agent and that, in fact, smallpox was widely considered the bioweapon agent of choice for some terrorist activities. And, importantly, it is not the only choice. Both the measles and polioviruses could be used as bioweapons, for example, as aerosols, the pathogenicity and transmission about which we know very little. Importantly, with the increasing accessibility of sophisticated molecular and bioengineering technology, all of these viruses could be genetically altered in ways that pose a tremendous challenge to post-eradication diagnosis and surveillance which, in order to be effective, must be able to detect novel viral variants; and to the vaccine industry which must be encouraged to continue research and development of new vaccines that offer protection against a constantly changing viral genome.

Accidental reintroduction from a stasis reservoir is also an important threat, as illlustrated by the 1977 re-emergence imputedly from frozen stock of a major variant of an influenza virus that had disappeared from circulation in the 1950s. Safe and secure biocontainment of the virus is essential for protecting both the environment and workers from accidental infection or contamination. Ensuring good biomanagement practices while simultaneously allowing legitimate and necessary viral research to continue presents a major challenge to post-eradication strategizing.

Although laboratory escape and the use of viruses for bioterrorism or biowarfare may be the most obvious sources of reintroduction in the post-eradication era, the evolution of new viral variants, reemergence from unknown zoonotic reservoirs, and reactivation from chronic carriers are equally important to consider. The rise of megacities and increasingly dense human populations and high-density animal feed lots provide favorable milieus for rapid microbial evolution. The creation of new reservoir hosts, cross-species transfer of infectious agents, rise of antimicrobial resistance, and immune evasion are all potential sources for the emergence of novel viral variants. Important and often overlooked, mass vaccination itself can also exert tremendous selective pressures and lead to the evolution of new infectious agents.

Even though no non-human reservoir has been identified for smallpox, polio, measles, or rubella, unknown non-human reservoirs may exist. The HIV pandemic is testament to the extraordinary clinical impact that a single zoonotic transmission event can have. In 2000, HIV-1 was estimated to have caused over 50 million infections worldwide.

Data show that humans are routinely exposed to a plethora of primate lentiviruses (SIVs) from which HIV is derived. Multiple incidents of zoonotic transmission of a virus create the potential for recombination between the human virus (e.g., HIV) and the newly introduced zoonotic virus (e.g., SIVs). If unknown non-human reservoirs are harboring variants or ancestors of the viruses responsible for disease, zoonotic transmissions may be a potential source for other viral diseases as well. Theoretical concerns about a non-human reservoir of measles, for example, raise questions about our assurance that the smallpox virus no longer resides in the natural environment. Given the rapid evolvability of viruses and the rapidly changing evolutionary pressures in a 21st-century world, it would not be surprising to see the gradual evolution of new, previously enzootic, diseases with human-to-human transmission properties.

Chronic carriers—HIV-infected persons, malnourished children, and other immunocompromised individuals—who can harbor and shed undetected virus for extended lengths of time are another important potential source of reemergence. More information is needed to better understand how long immunocompromised carriers continue to shed virus into the environment and what proportion of immunocompromised individuals shed virus for prolonged periods of time. This information is crucial to planning post-eradication vaccine production strategies, especially for polio. Because of its ability to revert to pathogenicity during replication in the gut, the oral, live-attenuated polio vaccine (OPV) used to prevent polio creates a serious challenge. OPV is usually shed from immunocompromised carriers for weeks to months but can be shed for as long as 10 years, compared to less than 3 months for immunocompetent carriers.

Indeed, the probability of genetic reversion from attenuation to pathogenicity must always be considered in the application of live-attenuated vaccines. As disease due to wild-type virus is eliminated, vaccine-associated cases become of increasing concern. Since 1973, the number of vaccine-associated paralytic poliomyelitis (VAPP) cases has exceeded the number of wild polio cases in the United States. Worldwide, there have been several epidemics caused by reversion of the polio vaccine to virulence, the most recent in 2000 in Hispaniola.

DETECTION AND SURVEILLANCE

Continued surveillance, improved surveillance methods, and assistance to lesser developed countries in their efforts to implement national surveillance campaigns are essential for the rapid detection of disease outbreaks. Given the biological variability of vaccine strains, and the innumerable array of samples in frozen storage, it is not a question of whether disease outbreaks will occur in the post-eradication era, but, rather, when and where.

Surveillance laboratory capacity must be strengthened, especially in areas where eradication has proven difficult to achieve or variants are likely to emerge. Surveillance tools must be sophisticated enough to detect different and new viral variants. To this end, global laboratory networks currently in place need to be further developed, especially for measles surveillance efforts. Measles surveillance is complicated by the fact that measles cases can be mistaken for dengue, rubella, scarlet fever, and roseola; thus, differential diagnosis based on clinical symptoms can be difficult, and laboratory surveillance is very important for detecting and reporting all cases. The measles laboratory network in the Americas is by far the most highly developed and should serve as a model for networks in other parts of the world.

National leaders must be convinced of the importance of strengthening surveillance capacity—not only to monitor the increasing likelihood of viral surprises as we enter a post-eradication era but also to more readily detect pockets of low immunity as eradication campaigns near completion. National surveillance programs must be strengthened and the WHO and able countries encouraged to provide support, as needed, to countries who do not already have national surveillance networks in place. To aid in this effort, revised International Health Regulations (IHR) will provide a template for core requirements for national surveillance systems in countries where they do not already exist. Ideally, the IHR revision process should involve broad consensus with all WHO member states; better working relationships among WHO, member states, and other international agencies whose work is related to the IHR need to be established.

The IHR are a set of global regulatory guidelines for how to respond to international disease threats and are currently the only binding set of regulations established on global surveillance for infectious diseases by WHO member states. They are designed to ensure maximum security against international spread of disease with minimum interference of world traffic and trade. However, the current IHR are limited in several ways; thus, the call for revision. Most importantly, they stipulate regulations for only three diseases, none of which are currently slated for eradication. The revised IHR will be more comprehensive and will apply to all "events of urgent international importance related to public health." An algorithm—or "decision tree"—is being developed for use in determining whether an event is of urgent, international public health importance.

Additionally, the current IHR regulations do not provide any mechanism for collaboration between member states and WHO. Even though the best way to prevent international spread of disease is to identify and stop local outbreaks before they begin to spread, national efforts often require international assistance. Such a conclusion recognizes the advantage of a single international entity (e.g., WHO) coordinating and overseeing global surveillance. Equally important, even local events can have international impact, especially if unauthorized information is disseminated in such a way that it causes overreaction and gratuitously damages tourism, traffic, or trade. Indeed, one of the motivations for revising IHR was the increasing threat of cross-border transmission due to increased transcontinental movement of people. The new IHR will require mechanisms to assure rapid communication between member states and WHO in the case of an outbreak; they will involve more collaboration between WHO and member states; and they will ensure the quick dissemination of information to appropriate sources.

Knowing if and when to discontinue surveillance in the post-eradication, post-immunization era poses a great challenge. With the continued threat of bioterrorism and reemergence of disease from unknown natural reservoirs or new viral variants, in combination with a decreased immunity and increased susceptibility in the population at large, it is likely that surveillance will need to be continued and strengthened even after immunization ceases, perhaps indefinitely. The potential usefulness of immunological surveillance—perhaps using a saliva antibody test to detect declining vaccination rates and pockets of susceptibility—as a supplement to disease surveillance needs to be further examined.

CONTINUED VIRAL RESEARCH IN THE POST-ERADICATION ERA

Although it may not seem worth arguing over whether a virus that only spreads among humans and has severe adverse health effects should be completely eliminated to the point of extinction, even in the laboratory, it may be necessary to retain samples for future study, especially given the rapid pace of viral evolution, the loss of immunity as infection disappears and immunization ceases, and the likelihood that new viral variants with altered pathogenicities or routes of transmission will emerge at some point in the post-eradication era. Too often, success or near-success at eliminating an infectious agent results in languished research efforts toward advancing knowledge of that agent.

In anticipation of polio eradication in the early 1990s, for example, polio research laboratories were told they would be soon required to cease poliovirus research and destroy all virus and infectious DNA stocks. The unfortunate consequence was that many research programs that could have contributed valuable information on new vaccines, new antiviral drugs, and animal models for virus transmission were shut down. If new vaccines or antiviral therapies are to be developed to cope with unforeseen viral challenges, basic scientific research on viral-host biology must continue even after eradication. Maintaining research programs that address important scientific questions about viral biology and pathogenesis will require an increased investment in containment laboratories and improved communication between the public health sector and research community.

Before viral stocks and samples can be safely contained, they need to be located. Inventories must include not only vials clearly labeled "measles" and "polio," for example, but also any biological samples, such as stool samples from patients who have had suspected enterovirus infections, that carry the risk of contamination. This is a daunting challenge. To complicate matters, many laboratories or clinics do not even realize that they have virus specimens until somebody stumbles upon them inadvertently.

Once identified, all viral stocks and samples should be transferred to biorepositories demonstrating well-developed and documented procedures for safe handling and security. This will ensure that the viruses are available for ongoing research, as needed, with a minimal risk of accidental reintroduction. Established standards, such as Biosafety Level 3 (BSL-3) and the more stringent BSL-4, have generally proven very successsful at protecting both workers and the environment from infection or contamination, where they have been in force. However, intermediate systems that incorporate more controls than BSL-3 but are not as stringent as BSL-4 often rely on ambiguous language and ill-defined protocol. Virus-specific standards need to be clearly established, based on known risks and properties unique to each virus.

Not only must virus stocks be safely contained in order to prevent accidental reintroduction, but precautions need to be taken to protect against intentional reintroduction as well. Internal security measures at biorepositories where the virus is housed should insure restricted physical access to the viruses (e.g., by securing freezers with locks that require two people to open), and freezer inventories should be designed in such a way that a locator code is needed to find the material. All movement of material should be tracked to verify authorized access. Only qualified end-users should be allowed access to the virus, and it must be assured that the receiving laboratory is capable of controlling access. End-users should demonstrate knowledge of the material and its potential hazards. Potential recipients should be screened by appropriate authorities, e.g., the departments of Commerce, State, and Treasury.

Undue proliferation of many regulations will hinder important scientific research. Restrictions may be necessary to prevent samples from falling into the "wrong hands," but the regime must acknowledge the need for scientific progress. It is imperative that the scientific and research community be proactive in presenting a reasonable framework for viral research to policy makers and legislators.

Physical containment of laboratory virus stock may become irrelevant with the advent of advanced recombinant and synthetic molecular technologies. Viral genes could readily be synthesized from nucleic acid sequences, and viruses themselves could probably be reconstituted from sequences or clones, thus precluding the need for continued storage of intact viruses. Importantly, however, individuals or organizations with bioterrorist intentions could do this just as well as legitimate research labs. And, as bioengineering technology advances, it becomes more possible to construct new, chimeric viruses. Although this would require greater planning, resources, and scientific expertise than simply removing intact stocks from a freezer, it may be an attractive alternative for persons or institutions with bioterrorist or biowarfare intentions. Although unlikely, the threat of a bioterrorist or biowarfare attack with an infectious agent of unknown properties reinforces the need to continue viral and antiviral research in support of improved vaccine and drug development.

VACCINES AND ANTIVIRAL THERAPIES FOR USE IN THE POST-ERADICATION ERA

Following eradication, smallpox vaccine production ceased in 1982. By the time it was realized that malevolent use of the smallpox virus posed a serious bioweapons threat and the Centers for Disease Control and Prevention (CDC) issued a contract for the production of a new national vaccine stockpile in 2000, the vaccine reserve was not only deficient but had decayed over time. The vaccine program infrastructure had deteriorated; vaccine technology used previously for smallpox vaccine production was outdated; and standards of vaccine production had changed.

In order for other disease post-eradication initiatives to avoid the type of catch-up campaign that production of the smallpox vaccine currently faces, vaccine production and research must continue even after immunization has ceased. This poses a tremendous challenge, as the financial incentives to develop and produce new vaccines are weak, and research leadership in this area is lacking. An in-date supply of vaccine must be made available for use in the event of an outbreak. Vaccine development must keep up with changing regulatory requirements, and improved vaccines must be able to protect against newly evolved or bioengineered viral strains with altered pathogenesis or routes of transmission. Stockpiles should be replenished regularly; expertise and experience of the manufacturing and control personnel should be maintained; and facilities, equipment, and the production process should be continually validated, as well as reliable means of storage. The size of vaccine stockpiles should correspond, at minimum, to the threshold immunity required to break transmission. New methods for rapid large-scale vaccine administration need to be developed and their immunogenicity demonstrated.

Given the tremendous success of vaccination in the prevention of infectious disease, one might question the necessity to develop other antiviral therapeutics. However, given the risk of reintroduction of disease, the evolvability of viruses, and the unknown changes that the human immune system will undergo against the background of zero immunity in the post-eradication era, other potentially useful antiviral strategies must be considered as means to strengthen the immune system or serve as adjuvant or prophylactic therapies.

Although diseases currently slated for eradication have never been considered targets for antiviral drug development, our knowledge of molecular biology and viral-host interactions has advanced to a point where selective, specific antiviral agents could be developed. Although broader-spectrum antiviral drugs, like interferon, would probably be more applicable (and more likely to attract investors) than narrowly focused drugs that only target specific viruses, they are notorious for their toxicity and many side effects; also, more research would be needed to identify host cell functions that could be targeted with a broader-spectrum antiviral drug. Although treatment with antivirals should never serve as a substitute for the prevention of disease, they can impact public health, as evident by their ability to reduce viral load in HIV-infected individuals. However, there are few incentives for manufacturers to invest in antiviral research, especially for vaccine-preventable diseases. If antiviral chemotherapy could be developed for a broad range of viral infections, it would drastically alter our assessment of risk of resurgence post-eradication.

Immunoprophylactics are another option. Although nonspecific immunoprophylactics (e.g., interferon) have been developed for treatment of a wide variety of diseases, experienced knowledge of toxicity and effectiveness of general prophylaxis against chronic infections in humans is very limited and would require extensive research before being considered for widespread use. Plus, given the readiness with which wild-type viruses evolve ways to escape host cell antiviral activities, it is unlikely that a universal prophylactic agent will be identified. More promising are prophylactic agents that target specific viruses. As with antivirals, the technology is now available to develop specific prophylactic agents against chronic infections like polio, measles, and rubella, but this has not been done.

Our approaches to disease prevention, mainly vaccination, rest upon the presumption that the human immune response has not changed for centuries and will remain strong for centuries to come, even as immunity changes in the post-eradication era. However, we do not know how true this is. In light of the possibility that our immune system may weaken in the post-eradication era—for example, from changing selective pressures—it would be a good idea to do all that we can to strengthen the immune response. Probiotic bacteria—living microbes introduced into the body to improve intestinal microbial balance—have great potential to sustain an immune response in the post-vaccine era and may prove useful in strengthening the immune response in immunocompromised individuals who are at risk for chronic infection. For example, recent studies have shown that probiotic lactobacilli can have a beneficial effect on the immune response in HIV-infected children.

It has long been understood that our human body space is shared with a multitude of microbial species, inhabiting our skin and mucous membranes. On the presumption that these may have varying effects on our health—from mutualistic enhancement through every grade of pathogenicity—we have been wont to regard them as a "microbiome", a collective set of genomes to be compared with our own intrinsic "human genome". As this is written, the day's headlines refer to studies regarding a protective effect of coinfection with the GBV-C, a relative of hepatitis-C virus, on the course of AIDS (Xiang et al., 2001; Tillmann et al., 2001). Proof is hard to find, but it makes evolutionary sense that any chronically infecting member of the microbiome would enhance its fitness by excluding the extinction of the host by more virulent competitors. In similar vein, we should not be surprised that Helicobacter secretes peptide antibiotics active against cholera, though there is not yet direct evidence that this has any clinical significance.

After eradication, the natural tendency is for vaccine and other relevant research funding—both public and private—to wither away. However, basic research on the immunological basis of protection will be vital to development of new vaccines and other antiviral therapeutics. A strong federally supported research program will be crucial to advancing our knowledge of viral genomics and pathogenesis in support of vaccine and antiviral drug development. Strong commitment is needed from both the public and private sectors to share the costs and risks associated with developing products which may have only a very short product life cycle. Research on non-vaccine antiviral therapies must be continued and strengthened in light of the fact that the post-eradication era may, ironically, pose even greater challenges to the immune system as immunity wanes and viruses evolve.

INSTITUTIONAL AND SYSTEMS PREPAREDNESS FOR DISEASE OUTBREAK

When discussing disease outbreaks in the post-eradication era, smallpox is of foremost concern since it is the only disease that has already been eradicated, plus we have a precedent for it. In 1946, in response to a new outbreak of smallpox and a single import from Mexico, six million New Yorkers were vaccinated. The question is, what would the situation be like if there were a recurrence of that same event today? First and foremost, would there be enough vaccine to vaccinate everyone who would need to be vaccinated? Who would need to be vaccinated? Where would the vaccine come from? And how would it be released? To complicate matters, today's population is much more susceptible to infection than it was in 1946, and emergency vaccination measures taken at that time were probably to some extent supererogatory since at least half of all New Yorkers were probably already vaccinated. It is likely that a newly introduced case would spread much more rapidly today than it would have done several decades ago.

Drawing on the lessons learned from smallpox eradication and as summarized above and discussed in detail throughout this report, a responsible post-eradication strategy must include provisions for vaccine reserves and contingency planning in case the disease re-emerges; continued surveillance and diagnostic activities; and research on and development of new vaccines and antiviral therapeutic drugs. The federal government will play a key role in supplying these provisions in the post-eradication era. With regard to vaccine production, for example, vaccines will become much less profitable to market after certification of eradication. Plus, over time, regulatory guidelines for vaccine manufacture are likely to become more troublesome as unforeseen safety issues arise (e.g., the risk of prion-mediated diseases resulting from incorporation of bovine derivatives into vaccines). Because of the increased cost of production and stricter regulatory guidelines, the private sector will likely lose interest in vaccine manufacture, and government-sponsored production may be necessary to maintain adequate vaccine supply.

The security consequences of a post-eradication oubreak should be assessed and prepared for from the outset of any eradication effort. Agents with biowarfare potential should be included in formal biological control negotiations, and information gathered to help determine if any nations or groups have sought to develop the agent as a bioweapon. The intelligence, arms control, law enforcement, and defense communities must be adequately prepared since they are all likely to be involved in the event of a disease outbreak with national security consequences. Intelligence information may be required to help determine if the outbreak was a natural or deliberate occurrence; evidence may need to be collected for legal or arms control issues; recurrence of disease outbreak will need to be prevented; and those responsible will need to be held accountable.

Hospitals serve as a major hub in the U.S. health care system and can and should play a major role in an outbreak response. However, at present, the U.S. health care system is not prepared to handle either a natural or intentional disease outbreak. It lacks the capacity and infrastructure; has neither incentives nor mandates that require preparedness; has no networks in place to aid in the coordination of response among different health care communities; and is plagued by unresolved staffing and legal policy issues. In order to effectively confront the demands of an outbreak, including the mass surge of people, the health care system must at least be operating effectively prior to the outbreak. However, U.S. hospitals are currently facing tremendous economic pressures, and current staff levels are insufficient to cope even with small and predictable influenza epidemics. Without funding incentives or mandates in place, it is unreasonable to expect that hospitals will take the necessary measures to prepare for disease outbreaks in the face of other, more pressing and immediate concerns.

Substantial communications barriers exist among and between public health agencies, emergency and first response communities, and medical care delivery communities. These barriers, combined with a climate of competition among hospitals and distrust across the public/private sector divide, prevent coordinated regional responses. Effective regional networks will require adequate funding, designation of an in-charge organization and individual, and development of a regional response plan.

The consequences of a disease outbreak in a post-eradication era will entail more than public health and security implications: the psychological response—particularly fear and panic—could hinder intervention and control. The media, government, and medical communities will play large roles in determining how the public will respond to an outbreak. While developing outbreak policies, the emotional and physical impact on leaders of these communities will need to be taken into account. Over-dedication, sleep deprivation, and the intensity of their roles during a crisis can lead to suboptimal decision-making and other manifestations of poor judgement. Protocols need to be developed for decision-making processes in the event of an outbreak. Research is needed on how to address the psychological and behavioral consequences of an outbreak, and the behavioral and societal effects of past infectious disease outbreaks should be studied in order to identify effects of different responses. Research is also needed on how best to enlist media support in the management of outbreaks, and risk communication programs need to be developed.

By definition, post-eradication outbreaks would involve infections rarely, if ever, seen in medical practice. Primary health care workers may have limited knowledge of the pathogen in question, making disease difficult to diagnose and treat. Untrained or mistrained responders could contribute to institutional breakdown. Poor medical knowledge can lead to conflicting messages and confusion regarding an appropriate course of action. While it is the nature of scientific discourse to debate and criticize, this will not instill confidence in a time of crisis and can lead to an undermining of authority. We need a better understanding of how the public should be trained to anticipate and cope with the diverse, and often conflicting, information that may be disseminated in the wake of an outbreak.

CONCLUSION

The current state of the U.S. health care system reveals a weakness in the United States' capacity to control outbreaks in a post-eradication era. However, this capacity is even weaker or even non-existent in poor countries who do not have any health infrastructure or resources to cope with an outbreak. Too often in the developing world, global eradication priorities override local health priorities. In the polio eradication effort, for example, countries have been pressured to focus on global priorities (to immunize everyone, for example, even if polio is not a disease that the people have witnessed) at the expense of eliminating other diseases that are killing their children but for which there is no global eradication effort. Recent reports indicate, however, that efforts to strengthen local health service infrastructures can operate synergistically with efforts to address global priorities—the two need not be mutually exclusive. In particular, evidence indicates that eradication efforts are more successful in countries with a strong health infrastructure in place. Focusing on building local health infrastructures and empowering communities with the resources to address their own problems in a self-reliant way is the best framework for dealing with disease outbreaks in a post-eradication era.

However, building local health infrastructure does not necessarily mean implementing the "doc-in-the-box" western model of primary health care centers. An important lesson learned from smallpox eradication was that vaccination could not be achieved by waiting for people to show up at a primary health care center. Rather, the vaccinators had to go out into the field and contact the people. Furthermore, what works in one locality may not work in another. Priorities for action must be based on an assessment of local resources and capabilities.

That so many countries still lack basic health services to prevent and cope with current public health crises, let alone capabilities to respond to a major disease outbreak in a post-eradication era, is indicative of the reality that even though post-eradication challenges need to be considered and prepared for concurrently with eradication efforts, still, except for smallpox, the post-eradication era may not be foreseeable in the near future. This is true even of polio, which is considered next in line for eradication. However optimistic we are about global eradication of polio, measles, rubella, or any other disease, current conditions in many parts of the world still pose significant challenges to eradication, let alone post-eradication strategizing.

There is some concern that too much focus on eradication, rather than on control, could divert resources and effort away from more pressing and serious public health crises. After all, the practice of good public health is based on the judicious and wise use of limited resources to achieve maximum public benefit; neither the international public health community nor any single nation has unlimited funds to support public health programs. Eradication is expensive, thus the decision to eradicate must be based on an in-depth review of all available funds and resources. Equally important, it must also be based on a thorough evaluation of the opportunities that may be lost by prioritizing actions and making decisions for the sake of eradication. For example, although polio is generally considered next in line for eradication, some participants in this workshop questioned the wisdom of focusing too much on polio eradication when there remain nearly a million people dying each year from measles. This high opportunity cost of polio eradication (i.e., lives lost) leads one to wonder if polio and measles eradication efforts should be conducted concurrently with more emphasis placed on controlling both, rather than eradicating one or the other. Another advantage to emphasizing control rather than eradication is that the former keeps us on guard that there might be still—somewhere on the planet—a threat great enough to motivate continued surveillance, vaccination, and research.

The information contained in this report provides important insights that can and should be incorporated into the decision-making process about whether to enter into future eradication efforts. With respect to polio eradication efforts, for example, a major selling point to political leaders was the potential post-eradication cost savings. But if we had known that immunization would likely need to be continued even in the post-eradication era, would the level of political commitment have been the same? If we had been more aware of the post-eradication challenges, would we have favored disease control rather than eradication and would development of the health infrastructure have been a better overall investment? These are difficult questions to ask. Many would contend that the eradication of smallpox is one of public health's greatest victories, a feat worthy of being emulated. Yet we must be cautious about embracing the ideology of eradication at the expense of sound, rational judgement. Given the challenges of managing the many post-eradication issues raised during this workshop, the public health community must consider all available evidence when deciding whether to launch similar efforts in the future.

Once a major disease has been eradicated, too much is at stake to return to a pre-eradication era. Post-eradication strategies need to be considered early on during an eradication campaign and developed when the possibility of eradication is certain. As population immunity wanes, viruses evolve, and complacency sets in, the catastrophic potential of a disease outbreak in the post-eradication era increases. It is crucial that we adequately prepare for recurrence of an outbreak, no matter how improbable. The issues raised in this workshop provide a framework for thinking about post-eradication policy and research needs that must be addressed now, before eradication of any other disease is certified and while there is still time to prepare and conduct crucial research that can influence how well we will meet the challenges of the post-eradication era.

REFERENCES

Tillmann HL, Heiken H, Knapik-Botor A, Heringlake S, Ockenga J, Wilber JC, Goergen B, Detmer J, McMorrow M, Stoll M, Schmidt RE, and Manns MP. 2001. Infection with GB virus C and reduced mortality among HIV-infected patients. *New England Journal of Medicine* 345(10):715–724.

Xiang J, Wunschmann S, Diekema DJ, Klinzman D, Patrick KD, George SL, and Stapleton JT. 2001. Effect of coinfection with GB virus C on survival among patients with HIV infection. *New England Journal of Medicine* 345(10):707–714.

1

Introduction

Ciro A. de Quadros, M.D., M.P.H.

Director, Division of Vaccines and Immunization
Pan American Health Organization, Washington, D.C.

HISTORY AND PROSPECTS FOR DISEASE ERADICATION

The concept of "disease eradication" originated in the late 18th century, when Edward Jenner inoculated James Phipps with the cowpox virus and subsequently infected him with the lethal smallpox virus. The inoculation protected Phipps from the smallpox, demonstrating the first successful vaccination against an infectious disease. Jenner concluded, "This practice would wipe out this scourge from the face of the earth" (Jenner, 1801).

Since then, eradication has been defined in many different ways. In 1997, the Dahlem Workshop on the Eradication of Infectious Diseases defined several levels of deliberate efforts of disease control, including eradication, as follows (Dowdle and Hopkins, 1998):

- *Control*: reduction of disease incidence, prevalence, morbidity, and mortality to acceptable levels;
- *Elimination of disease*: reduction to zero incidence of disease in a defined geographic area;
- *Elimination of infection*: reduction to zero incidence of infection caused by a specific agent in a defined geographic area;
- *Eradication*: permanent reduction to zero worldwide incidence of infection caused by a specific agent;
- *Extinction*: the specific agent no longer exists in nature or the laboratory.

The first three levels of disease control require that intervention measures be continued in order to reduce and prevent reestablishment of transmission. Once eradication and/or extinction are/is achieved, intervention measures can be discontinued.

These definitions were debated at the Conference on Global Disease Elimination and Eradication as Public Health Strategies in Atlanta, Georgia, in February, 1998. There was no consensus on the proposed definitions, so a small group convened after the conference to continue the debate. The group concluded that because the terms elimination and eradication were synonymous in many languages, thus they proposed that elimination be discontinued with subsequent use of the following three levels of deliberate efforts at disease control:[1]

- *Control*: the reduction of disease in a defined geographic area; intervention measures cannot be discontinued;
- *Eradication:* the absence of a disease agent in nature in a defined geographic area; control measures can be discontinued once the risk of importation of the agent is no longer present;
- *Extinction*: the specific disease agent no longer exists in nature or the laboratory.

With these definitions, the term eradication can be used in different geographic levels, such as "eradication of a disease in a given area or country," "eradication from a region or regions of the world," and, ultimately, the "eradication of a disease globally."

PRECONDITIONS FOR DISEASE ERADICATION

Several preconditions must be met before eradication can be considered. These include biological characteristics of the infectious agent, as well as various social and political factors outlined by the 1997 Dahlem Workshop (Dowdle and Hopkins, 1998):

- The microbial agent can infect only humans.
- There cannot be a non-human reservoir for the microbial agent.
- The infection must induce life-long immunity.
- There must be a tool or intervention that effectively interrupts the chain of transmission of the infectious agent from one individual to another.

[1]These definitions reflect the author's experience and are not necessarily consistent with those of other authors contributing to this book.

- There must be political committment in the form of sufficient human and financial resources to carry the initiative from beginning to end.
- The burden of disease must be considered of great public health importance with broad international impact.

HISTORY: SUCCESSES AND FAILURES

Past major attempts at disease eradication are noted in Table 1-1. Not included in Table 1-1 is the 1909 initiative of Dr. C. W. Stiles, U.S. Public Health Service, with support by the Rockefeller Foundation, to interrupt hookworm transmission in the southern United States. This effort was later expanded to 56 countries in 6 continents and 29 island groups. Other initiatives not included are those aimed at the eradication of other helminthic diseases and those aimed at disease vectors, such as the successful Soper initiative to eradicate *Anopheles gambiae* from Brazil and the failed attempt to eradicate *Aedes aegypti* from the Americas.

Yellow fever eradication efforts failed majorly because the disease did not fulfill the biological preconditions for eradication: yellow fever has a non-human reservoir (i.e., it is transmitted by mosquitoes).

Smallpox was the first globally eradicated disease. Smallpox eradication was an extraordinary initiative which set the example for future disease eradication programs. The smallpox eradication program was initially based on the premise that mass vaccination campaigns would stop transmission, but the program managers soon recognized that this strategy was not sufficient to achieve the objective. Cases of smallpox continued to occur in areas of the world reporting very high immunization coverage. Therefore, in 1967 the focus of the program switched from vaccination alone to

TABLE 1-1 Major Attempts at Disease Eradication

Year	Program Leader	Program (Location)
1801	Edward Jenner	Smallpox (Global)
1911	William Gorgas	Yellow Fever (Americas)
1915	Rockefeller Commission	Yellow Fever (Global)
1950	Fred Soper	Smallpox (Americas)
1954	WHO	Yaws (Regional)
1955	WHO	Malaria (Global)
1958	Viktor Zhdanov	Smallpox (Global)
1985	PAHO	Polio (Americas)
1986	WHO	Guinea Worm (Global)
1988	WHO	Polio (Global)
1994	PAHO	Measles (Americas)

a two-pronged effort combining vaccination with surveillance and containment.

The main lesson to be learned from the success of smallpox eradication is that all of the preconditions for disease eradication were met:

- All biological conditions for disease eradication were fulfilled.
- There was an effective tool available for interrupting the chains of transmission (i.e., an effective heat-stable vaccine easily administered with a bifurcated needle).
- Endemic countries were politically committed to the effort.
- The strategy was clearly understood at all levels.
- Resources were made available when required.
- Strong management was present at all levels.
- Continuing research was available to guide the strategy.
- Adequate international coordination supported program operations.
- International and national staff were highly motivated to see the program succeed.

LESSONS FROM RECENT EXPERIENCES: POLIO AND MEASLES ERADICATION IN THE AMERICAS

The lessons learned from smallpox eradication were subsequently applied to the Pan American Health Organization (PAHO) initiatives to eradicate both poliomyelitis and measles from the Americas.

Polio

The polio eradication initiative was launched in May 1985, with the goal of interrupting transmission of the disease by the end of 1990. The strategy was based on the initial proposals of Albert Sabin, who suggested that polio transmission could be interrupted if the oral polio vaccine (OPV) were administered simultaneously to a large number of children (i.e., under five years of age) in a very short period of time (i.e., in one day or week). The effectiveness of this strategy was demonstrated in Cuba in the early 1960s, where transmission was stopped after the first two rounds of national immunization days (NIDs). In 1980, Brazil initiated a similar program which had a tremendous positive impact on polio incidence after the first few rounds of NIDs.

Thus, the eradication strategy in the Americas relied on biannual NIDs held at least four weeks apart. OPV was administered to all children under five years of age as a supplement to routine vaccinations administered by each country's health system infrastructure.

Surveillance was a key component of the program from day one. However, countries free of poliomyelitis when the program was launched did not want to report cases of suspect poliomyelitis; they were concerned that the reports would affect tourism. So surveillance targeted acute flaccid paralysis (AFP) instead. A small network of laboratories—nine for the entire region—was established for the purpose of investigating clinical cases of AFP and determining if any were due to the infection with the wild poliovirus. The labs were closely supervised and subject to routine quality control.

There were four pieces of information gathered during implementation of the initiative that proved critical to the program's success. First, the surveillance network that targeted AFP was expanded from an initial 500 to over 20,000 sites, covering every district in each country. The initial network of reporting units primarily involved main hospitals and rehabilitation clinics. But when it was learned that patients were seeking initial care in the peripheral health units before eventually being referred to the tertiary care level, the reporting unit networks were extended to include these peripheral health units as well because by the time patients arrived at hospitals and rehabilitation clinics, it was usually too late for the appropriate collection of stools necessary for identification of the virus.

Second, the analysis of epidemiological data that had accumulated over the first couple of years indicated that in the absence of wild poliovirus, cases of AFP occurred at a rate of at least one case per 100,000 persons under 15 years of age. This rate became one of the primary indicators of a country's compliance with adequate surveillance.

Third, as the program was winding down in Brazil, an outbreak of poliovirus type-3 was detected. Analysis of the outbreak indicated that the composition of the trivalent vaccine did not contain adequate quantities of poliovirus type-3; therefore, the manufacturers were asked to reformulate the vaccine. This highlights the need to constantly reevaluate and improve the tools available for disease control.

Fourth, despite high immunization coverage during NIDs, cases continued to occur in several countries. The empiric observation that outbreaks of polio would always originate in the same areas of a given country and subsequently spread to other parts of the country indicated that the polioviruses remained in certain reservoirs during periods of low incidence. This observation was confirmed by molecular epidemiology from Dr. Olen Kew and his colleagues, who determined the geographical distribution of different genotypes of the three polioviruses types in the region. These findings were applied to the program strategy and allowed for complementing NIDs with "mopping-up" operations in the main reservoirs of the disease. The introduction of these operations enhanced immunity in those reservoirs and interrupted the last chains of transmission.

The ways by which these four pieces of information fed back into the program strategy demonstrate the need to constantly analyze information generated in the field in order to adjust eradication strategies.

The global polio eradication initiative is based on lessons learned from polio eradication in the Americas. However, global implementation of all of the various components of the strategy proven so effective in the Americas has been very slow. Surveillance was introduced very late in the program, and only recently have mopping-up operations been included as an essential part of program operations. These tactical mistakes, coupled with the lack of funds and civil unrest in many endemic countries, accounts for the delay in completion of the global program.

Measles

After the Americas region was certified polio-free in September 1994, the PAHO Directing Council launched an initiative to eradicate measles from the Americas by the year 2000. The measles vaccine had been introduced in most countries of the region in the 1980s and had been used simultaneously with OPV during NIDs. It was no surprise, therefore, that by the time polio was declared eradicated, measles incidence was low. In fact, Cuba and the English-speaking Caribbean had already launched measles eradication programs. Cuba started its major campaign against measles in 1987, and the English-speaking Caribbean in 1990—both with a very high degree of success in interrupting indigenous transmission.

The strategy for interrupting measles transmission was based on changes in the epidemiology of the disease after the vaccine had been introduced. In the pre-vaccine era, all children contracted measles at an early age; by age five, nearly 90% of all children had contracted the disease. Disease outbreaks occurred every one and a half to two years, as new cohorts of susceptible children were introduced into the population. As the outbreaks occurred, the population of susceptibles diminished and the disease subsided, until a new cohort of susceptibles again fueled transmission of the infectious agent.

With the introduction of vaccine, measles epidemiology changed radically. Epidemics began to occur less frequently, depending on the level of coverage in a country. In some countries, several years may elapse between epidemics. As a result, some groups of children remain susceptible into adulthood, thus the incidence of disease has increased among older children and young adults.

Another important criteria for developing a measles eradication strategy was vaccine effectiveness. Measles vaccine is only about 90–95% effective when administered to children older than 12 months. Therefore, it was expected that even in programs achieving high vaccination coverage using either one or two doses, many children would still fail to sero-convert to an immune status.

Given these considerations, the strategy used in Cuba and the English-speaking Caribbean—and subsequently applied in all other Latin American countries—aimed at interrupting the chains of transmission among those most affected by the disease. Analysis of attack rates by age group indicated that in most Latin American countries, the majority of measles cases occurred in children under 15 years of age.

The recommended PAHO strategy relied initially on four main components:

1. A one-time-only mass campaign conducted in a very short period of time during the low season for disease transmission and aimed at vaccinating all children between one and fourteen years of age with one dose of measles-containing vaccine (either M, MR, or MMR) was recommended. These "catch-up" campaigns generally achieve 90–95% coverage of the target population.
2. Maintenance of a routine measles vaccination program aimed at vaccinating all new birth cohorts immediately after these children reach 12 months of age was recommended. These "keep-up" vaccination programs generally target 90–95% coverage.
3. Since many children who are not vaccinated or fail to sero-convert remain susceptible into adulthood, mass "follow-up" campaigns targeting all children between one and four years of age were recommended every four years. The interval of four years was decided by taking into account the coverage achieved in most countries in the Americas: given the present 80–90% level of coverage for children between twelve and twenty-four months of age, it takes approximately four years for the susceptible population to grow to a point where it could fuel an epidemic if the virus were ever introduced into the population.
4. Surveillance should be simple and sensitive enough to detect cases of fever and rash disease in all situations where health workers suspect measles. This requires that trained epidemiologists investigate suspected cases, and blood specimens be collected for laboratory testing. This activity has been supported by the establishment of a network of laboratories dedicated to performing serological tests and virus isolation.

The results from the measles campaign have been very successful. Measles transmission is believed to be interrupted in most countries of the Americas. Only 1,500 cases—the lowest number ever reported for this region—were reported during 2000.

The first lesson from this initiative is that the administration of an injectable vaccine that does not immunize early after birth can be used to interrupt disease transmission. The second lesson is that while measles transmission has been curtailed in the region, most cases are now imported from the industrialized countries of Europe and Asia, for example France, Germany, Italy, and Japan.

A third lesson relates to the economics of measles eradication. A recent cost-effectiveness study (Arnab et al., submitted for publication) of measles eradication in the Americas shows that while the extra expenditure to achieve interruption of transmission has been approximately $240 million over the last six years, approximately $430 million has been saved in treatment costs. Like the eradication of smallpox and polio, the eradication of measles will be a major cost-saving operation for the health sector.

The fourth lesson refers to the impact of fever and rash surveillance on detecting the burden of other diseases. For example, as soon as measles disappeared from most countries, rubella was identified as a major public health problem. Some countries are now planning to interrupt rubella transmission as a first step toward eradication of rubella and its serious sequelae, congenital rubella syndrome (CRS). This has already been achieved in Cuba and several areas of the English-speaking Caribbean, and is now being attempted in Chile and Costa Rica. The strategies being used for rubella eradication are based on the lessons learned from measles eradication.

Success of Polio and Measles Eradication in the Americas

The efforts toward polio and measles eradication in the Americas have been possible only because the diseases meet the main preconditions for eradication outlined previously. Notably, there was a very high level of political commitment and collaboration among governments of the region and a very effective collaboration between regional governments and the international agencies involved.

Intra-regional collaboration, which rose to levels never achieved previously, has helped strengthen other regional initiatives, such as joint purchases of vaccines through a PAHO revolving fund. It has also accelerated control of other diseases, such as neo-natal tetanus, and the launching of other disease eradication initiatives. For example, at the end of the first day of polio immunizations during the three-day campaign to halt the vaccine-derived polio outbreak in the Dominican Republic in December 2000, the government of the Dominican Republic realized that there would be vaccine shortage in view of the high campaign turn-out. A direct call between the ministries of health of the Dominican Republic and Haiti resulted in 400,000 doses of OPV being driven across the border from Haiti within eight hours, ensuring successful vaccination of 1.2 million children under five years of age. Subsequently, in January 2001, the Dominican Republic lent 1,000 thermoses to Haiti to facilitate the logistics of vaccine distribution during their polio campaign.

The availability of resources for both the polio and measles eradication initiatives was partly contingent on the establishment of an operational timeline for completion. Such operational timelines are important for all disease eradication programs to prevent the institutional fatigue that would develop within governments and collaborating partners when timely objectives are not met or cannot be measured for success.

A final lesson from the polio and measles eradication efforts in the Americas is that the polio eradication effort in particular had a very positive impact on strengthening the health systems/services infrastructure. This is well documented by a study conducted in several countries in the Americas by the Commission on the Impact of the Expanded Program on Immunization and the Polio Eradication Initiative on Health Systems in the Americas, chaired by Dr. Carl Taylor (PAHO, 1995).

PROSPECTS FOR ERADICATION OF OTHER VIRAL DISEASES

The 1998 Conference on Global Disease Elimination and Eradication as Public Health Strategies concluded that there are three viral diseases besides polio that are potentially eradicable at this time, provided that all preconditions outlined above are met. These diseases are hepatitis A, measles, and rubella.

The conference participants concluded that other viral zoonotic diseases, such as yellow fever, rabies, and Japanese encephalitis are not eradicable at this time because their infectious agents all have non-human reservoirs. Nor are influenza, mumps, and varicella, even though they all have available vaccines. Eradication of influenza virus is impeded by its antigenic instability, frequent mutations, and regular reassortment with influenza virus circulating through birds and livestock, all of which contribute to the need for constant reformulation of the vaccine. Although mumps may be biologically eradicable, the low priority accorded to this disease makes it operationally unfeasible for eradication. Finally, the long-term carrier state among herpes zoster-infected individuals suggests that eradication of varicella is not feasible.

Even though the disease is considered eradicable at this time, hepatitis A virus eradication efforts face considerable impeding factors. The hepatitis A vaccine is costly and cannot be used in infancy or early childhood. Further research is needed to develop a hepatitis A vaccine formulation for use in children under two years of age.

The major impeding factor for rubella is the societal feasibility of rubella eradication. The burden of rubella, particularly of CRS, is not well known in most developing countries.

As global eradication of polio nears completion, measles becomes the next target for global eradication. Eradication strategies developed in the Americas have proven effective in interrupting transmission among large geographic areas for long periods of time. Even in the presence of imported cases, transmission has not been reestablished in those countries fully implementing the strategy. However, a major inhibiting factor is that measles is not perceived as a priority in the industrialized world. Plus, the health infrastructure among developing countries is not strong enough to maintain high vaccination coverage in all birth cohorts, which means that the required frequency of mass immunization campaigns is high and the associated cost enormous.

CONCLUSION

The global eradication of smallpox, the eradication of poliomyelitis from the Americas and its near-global eradication, and the near-eradication of measles from the Americas demonstrate the tremendous progress achieved in disease eradication efforts.

However, the recent outbreak of poliomyelitis in the Americas caused by vaccine-derived poliovirus type-1 suggests caution in determining when to launch eradication initiatives. The interruption of wild poliovirus transmission in the Americas and other parts of the world has relied heavily on the use of oral live-attenuated polio vaccines which have a long history of safety and effectiveness. Although it has been known for many years that live-attenuated vaccines can revert to virulence, this fact has always been considered of little epidemiological significance. In 1964, for example, Wilna Woods and Fred Robbins wrote in the *American Journal of Hygiene* that, "The remote possibility exists that a vaccinee, at any particular time, might be excreting a virulent strain. The large amount of evidence that has been accumulated concerning the safety of type 1 vaccine virus would indicate that this is not a matter of any great practical importance" (Woods et al., 1964).

Although the occurrence of this phenomenon in Hispaniola is a rare event and has been observed only twice before, in Egypt and China, advances in science—from the monkey virulence test of the 1960s to the genetic sequencing of viruses—are providing newer perspectives on how to deal with these problems. Undoubtedly, the vaccine-derived outbreak in Hispaniola will make the discontinuation of control measures much more difficult, especially once wild polioviruses are eradicated from the world. As previously defined, "Eradication is the absence of a disease agent in nature in a defined geographic area, and control measures can be discontinued once the risk of importation is no longer present." Therefore, while it is important that we accelerate activities aimed at the final interruption of wild poliovirus transmission in the world, it is also important that we accelerate research on the optimal strategy for the final discontinuation of polio vaccination.

By removing a major health threat, eradication of disease provides one of the greatest health benefits for humankind. It is the quintessential example of health equity, as all humankind reaps the benefits and it allows for immeasurable cost savings. In the future, the biotechnology revolution will likely yield numerous new vaccines, even for diseases considered chronic and degenerative, thus it is very important that we continue to search for those diseases that could eventually be eradicated. As Louis Pasteur pointed out, "It is within the power of man to eradicate infection from the earth" (Dubos and Dubos, 1953).

REFERENCES

Arnab A, Diaz-Ortega JL, Tambini G, de Quadros CA, and Arita A. Cost-effectiveness of measles eradication in Latin America and the Caribbean: a prospective analysis. Submitted for publication, 2001.

Dowdle WR and Hopkins DR, eds. 1998. *The Eradication of Infectious Diseases* (Report of the Dahlem Workshop on the Eradication of Infection Diseases, Berlin, March 16–22, 1997). New York: John Wiley & Sons.

Dubos R and Dubos J. 1953. The White Plague: Tuberculosis, Man, and Society. London: Gollancz.

Jenner E. 1801. The Origin of the Vaccine Innoculation. London: D.N. Shury.

PAHO (Pan American Health Organization). 1995. The Impact of the Expanded Program on Immunization and the Polio Eradication Initiative on Health Systems in the Americas. Report of the Taylor Commission. Washington, DC: PAHO.

Woods WA, Robbins FC, Weiss RA, Cashel J, and Kirschstein RL. 1964. Characteristics of sabin type 1 poliovirus after gastrointestinal passage in newborn infants. *The American Journal of Hygiene* 79(2):236–244.

2

Major Efforts for Disease Eradication

OVERVIEW

The eradication of smallpox is the only successful global eradication campaign thus far and is testament to the immeasurable public health benefits that can be achieved through eradication. There is optimism that several other viral diseases are candidates for global eradication in the near future given sufficient resources, effort, and international cooperation. These include, in their order of likely eradication, polio, measles, and rubella, all of which satisfy the necessary preconditions for eradication. However, there were many factors that uniquely favored smallpox eradication, and each of these other diseases involves major challenges which must be overcome before eradication can be achieved.

Major lessons learned from the global smallpox eradication program are that the necessary vaccination technology must be in hand and the practicality of eradication must be demonstrated in the field before eradication can be considered. Lack of preparation invites costly failure and, more importantly, the loss of credibility for public health professionals who are leading the initiatives.

Data from the Americas show that measles transmission can be interrupted on entire continents; thus, eradication is technically feasible. Lack of sufficient political will is probably the greatest impediment to global measles eradication. Some of the lowest measles vaccine coverage rates occur in the richest countries. The industrialized world must be encouraged to increase vaccine coverage in order to reduce the likelihood of their becoming reservoirs for the virus and to increase their funding to developing countries where measles takes its greatest toll. Measles results in approximately 900,000 deaths per year, half of which occur in Africa.

Likewise, eradication of rubella by correct application of a measles-rubella or measles-mumps-rubella vaccine is feasible. However, a major challenge to congenital rubella syndrome (CRS) eradication are inapparent, or subclinical, infections which make diagnosis and surveillance very difficult. CRS eradication efforts are also encumbered by a general lack of awareness of the disease.

Polio has been regionally eradicated from the Americas (the last indigenous case was in 1991) and is expected to be the next globally eradicated infectious viral disease. Once eradicated, knowing if, how, and when to stop immunization will be a major challenge. Cessation of immunization will require assurance that OPV-derived viruses are no longer circulating and that laboratory poliovirus stocks are adequately contained.

SMALLPOX

D.A. Henderson, M.D., M.P.H.

Director, Center for Civilian Biodefense Studies
The Johns Hopkins University, Baltimore, MD

The eradication of smallpox removed, hopefully forever, one of the greatest of all the world's plagues. With a 30% fatality rate, smallpox was in a class by itself as a global health problem. Eradication was an extraordinary, cooperative effort involving, under World Health Organization (WHO) leadership, countries throughout the world and perhaps as many as 150,000 field staff at various points during the campaign (Fenner et al., 1988). It dramatically demonstrated the extraordinary cost-benefit ratios that might be achieved with eradication. The total investment in international assistance was just under $100 million; national investments were estimated to be perhaps $200 million. Yet, because vaccination and quarantine measures are no longer necessary, savings of at least $1 billion annually are being realized.

Lessons for Eradication of Other Diseases

Poliomyelitis is generally considered to be the next candidate for eradication, and a heroic effort is now being made to eradicate it. However, given the task yet to be done and the many current uncertainties, it would be presumptuous to forecast a reasonably certain date for polio eradication, its status now being roughly where we were with smallpox some five years before transmission was finally stopped. Thus, as the first lesson from the smallpox campaign, and before indulging in extended discussions about what might or might not be done post-eradication, it would be productive to ascertain whether, in the cold hard light of accumulating experience and available technology, there are reasonable prospects for the eradication of any other disease within the next ten to twenty years.

So far, there have been seven campaigns intended to eradicate an infectious disease globally. The first four failed; only one—smallpox—succeeded; and two are still in progress. Despite the fact that there has been only one success in eradicating a disease, many experts speculate that a wide variety of diseases and conditions should be susceptible to eradication given sufficient resources, effort, and cooperation. However, this is precisely the wrong lesson to be learned from the smallpox campaign.

There were many factors that uniquely favored smallpox eradication:

- No other disease has features that made diagnosis and surveillance for infection so easy. Because every infected person had a characteristic rash, the presence or absence of the virus could be determined quickly in every geographic area.
- Most transmission was through droplets spread by face-to-face contact, making outbreak containment comparatively easy.
- It was one of the few diseases that both confers permanent immunity and has no carrier state or animal reservoir (two important preconditions for the eradication of disease—see Chapter 1).
- The smallpox vaccine had many advantageous properties: it was heat-stable and inexpensive; it provided protection with only a single inoculation, it could be administered anytime from birth onward; and, using the new bifurcated needle, vaccination was simply accomplished.

Given the fact that all countries were deeply concerned about smallpox and were regularly vaccinating large numbers of their citizens, it was an eradication program that should have commanded the highest possible political commitment. However, expected voluntary contributions to the program were sparse at best, and inadequate funds seriously hampered the program throughout its first nine years of existence. A number of endemic countries had to be cajoled into undertaking any program at all. On several occasions, the program hung in the balance because of political and social problems and, despite the best efforts of technical staff, could well have suffered serious setbacks that delayed eradication, perhaps indefinitely. Not until seven years into the program were the staff confident that eradication could be achieved, and events as late as 12 months prior to the last case threatened a successful conclusion.

Vaccine played an especially critical role in the success of the smallpox program. The smallpox vaccine had been known since 1798, but not until the end of the 19th century did large quantities become available as a result of growth of the virus on the flank of cows. Transporting it, however, was a problem. Thus, smallpox continued to spread largely unabated in most of the world, except in industrialized countries where sufficiently rapid transport and refrigeration were possible. Finally, in Indonesia in the 1930s, a vaccine that retained potency for periods of six months or more at 37°C was perfected by air-drying over sulfuric acid. Although often heavily contaminated, take rates of 80%+ were usual. By the end of the 1930s, Indonesia was smallpox-free. A similar product was introduced into a number of French colonies with similarly dramatic results.

In 1967, when the global smallpox campaign began, there were a number of Latin American, east Asian, and African countries where smallpox transmission had been stopped. This was due in large part to the use of the air-dried vaccine or a new freeze-dried product developed in the early 1950s.

Thus, vaccine technology had advanced to the point where eradication was a feasible proposition. Had we been dependent on a vaccine no more heat-stable nor immunogenic than, for example, polio vaccine, the prospects for eradication would have been significantly diminished.

Post-Eradication Strategies

During the course of the eradication campaign, there was very little planning for post-eradication strategies and activities. Procedures were developed for certifying large contiguous geographic areas as smallpox-free, but this was the extent of the effort. In major part, this reflected the belief that the margin for error in the program was small and that all available resources had to be directed toward the goal of interrupting smallpox transmission. Otherwise, there would be no post-eradication era. In fact, transmission continued for one year beyond the date anticipated, when smallpox invaded Somalia, spread throughout the country, and threatened the whole of the Middle East. Not until late 1975, when smallpox was confined to Ethiopia, and the interruption of transmission appeared to be only a matter of months away, were significant efforts made to define post-eradication needs.

In December 1979, the Global Commission for the Certification of Smallpox Eradication, as part of its final report, made 19 recommendations for post-eradication actions (WHO, 1980). The recommendations were subsequently approved by the 1980 World Health Assembly (WHA), after which a special committee, the Orthopoxvirus Committee, regularly met every four years up until recently. Some of the post-eradication actions taken in response to the recommendations are described below.

Vaccine and Vaccination (Recommendations 1–6)

Most countries discontinued routine vaccination by 1982, and all countries by 1984. By that time, countries had also stopped requiring travelers to show certificates of proof of recent smallpox vaccination. A few countries continued to vaccinate their military, but that practice ceased by about 1990.

Seed lot vials of smallpox vaccine were produced at the Rijks Institute (The Netherlands) and distributed to several vaccine production centers for storage to assure that vaccinia virus would be available at several sites, should it ever be needed. Vaccine was also stored in rented cold storage lockers at two locations in Switzerland and regularly retitered to assure that it retained potency, which it did. But the costs of vaccine storage and periodic retitering were considerable, and WHO budgets were under great stress due in large part to the U.S. failure to pay its assessments to the organization. Thus, in 1990, nearly 13 years after the last known case, the committee recommended, perhaps prematurely, that the WHO stockpile be reduced from 200 million doses to 500,000 doses, and that the balance of the vaccine be sent back to its respective donor countries. As of 1999, individual countries reported retaining as much as 80 million doses of vaccine, not all of which has been properly stored or retitered.

Suspect Cases of Smallpox (Recommendations 7, 8)

As anticipated, rumors of possible smallpox cases continued to be reported to WHO. It was considered important that all rumors be thoroughly investigated so as to provide assurance to the international community that there were no further naturally occurring cases. The number of rumors decreased from 30 or so annually in the first two years to 10 per year by 1985, with a scattering of cases thereafter. About half were found to be chickenpox or measles, one-third were erroneous news reports, and the rest, a miscellaneous collection of skin diseases.

Laboratory Retention of Specimens (Recommendations 9–15)

A major concern following eradication was the possible reintroduction of smallpox virus from a laboratory. Limiting the number of laboratories that retained smallpox virus was considered an important step in mitigating the risk of this occurring. In 1975, a survey was undertaken to determine which laboratories might have retained smallpox isolates. All countries and 823 laboratories included in the WHO list of virus laboratories were contacted. Special contacts were made with those laboratories that had published papers over the preceding 25 years indicating that they had grown smallpox virus. A total of 75 laboratories, nearly two-thirds of which were in Europe and the Americas, reported having smallpox virus isolates in 1975.

The comparatively small number of labs is explained by the fact that most virus labs did not process smallpox virus specimens:

- Clinical characteristics were sufficient for diagnosis, and laboratory confirmation was seldom required.
- Growth on chick chorioallantoic membrane (CAM) was necessary for diagnosis and, in many areas, suitable uncontaminated eggs were extremely difficult to obtain.
- Laboratory researchers preferred to work with other orthopoxviruses for which there were suitable animal models for infection.
- The need for many countries to develop their own laboratories was diminished because official WHO Collaborating Laboratories provided laboratory services.

Following a request by the WHA that the laboratories destroy their isolates or transfer them to one of the two WHO Collaborating Laboratories, 57 of the 75 reported that they had done so by July 1977. No effort was made by WHO to confirm these reports. It was recognized that laboratories customarily retain microbial isolates for later reference, and that such specimens were not always well-referenced. A search of all deep freezers in the relevant laboratories throughout the world was far beyond the resources of WHO. The objective of mitigation of risk of release of smallpox virus was as much as could be reasonably expected.

In 1978, a laboratory-associated outbreak in Birmingham, England, prompted a number of countries to destroy or transfer isolates to WHO laboratories. By 1980, only six laboratories reported holding the virus but they strenuously resisted parting with specimens. However, by 1983, WHO had reduced this number to two. Both labs were regularly inspected by WHO consultants.

In 1994, the WHO Orthopoxvirus Committee, in a report to the Director General, recommended that the 1995 WHA pass a resolution calling for the destruction of all remaining stocks of smallpox virus in June 1995. By that time, representative strains of variola virus had been prepared as a cloned fragment library and sequenced. A five-year study of monkeypox demonstrated it to be a zoonotic virus which only occasionally infected humans and which was unable to sustain human-to-human transmission (Jezek and Fenner, 1988). No research was known to have been conducted using smallpox virus for at least the past 12 years. In fact, the virus was known to have been grown only at the Centers for Disease Control and Prevention (CDC) to produce material for sequencing and to validate diagnostic tests. The WHO laboratory in Moscow ceased research in 1982 and, in a later written report, Dr. Sandakhchiev, Director of the Novosibirsk Laboratory to which the Moscow strains had been sent, asserted that they had undertaken no laboratory studies using variola virus until July 1996. At that time, the only stated reason for retaining the virus was a hypothetical one—perhaps some day, someone would wish to undertake some type of research that would require the intact variola virus. Weighing the risks associated with retaining it against a hypothetical scientific need, the committee, supported by five major scientific societies that had been explicitly consulted, recommended its destruction.

As concerns grew about the use of smallpox as a biological weapon, scientists from a number of nations argued that the virus should be retained for research purposes to develop an anti-viral drug or improved vaccine. It was generally recognized that to do so would be costly and, even if a product were produced, its effectiveness in humans could not be determined. In 1999, WHA delegates voted to defer a final decision on the destruction of the virus until 2002. Additionally, the United States contracted for 40 million vaccine doses to be produced for use in an emergency.

What Lessons Does the Smallpox Eradication Experience Provide?

- Disease eradication is extremely difficult even when, as in the case of smallpox, the disease is severe, a heat-stable, highly effective single-dose vaccine is available, and the epidemiological characteristics are as close to ideal as one might wish.
- The direct implications of a failed eradication program can be significant. For most diseases, the cost of eradication is far greater than that of control (see Chapter 1 for definitions of eradication and control). Unless eradication is achieved within a finite time, and control measures can be stopped or significantly decreased, the added costs of eradication will not be recouped. Moreover, experience has shown that failed eradication programs in most areas, although resulting in better control while special measures are in place, gradually revert to a pre-eradication status as special funds and interest fade.
- For sometime after the declaration of eradication, the only likely sources for the reintroduction of smallpox virus were from victims exhumed from the tundra or escape from the laboratory. In either case, it was felt that the outbreaks would be small and readily containable. Use of smallpox as a biological weapon was considered to be unlikely, but potentially catastrophic if outbreaks were to occur. The fact that the Soviet Union, during the 1980s, had engaged in a massive research and development program to produce smallpox virus as a biological weapon heightened this concern.

- Persuading most laboratories to destroy or transfer smallpox virus to WHO Collaborating Laboratories posed few problems. A few objected strongly, and cooperation was achieved only with difficulty. In 1999, the WHA, passed unanimously a resolution which reads as follows: "1) Strongly reaffirms the decision of previous Assemblies that the remaining stocks of variola virus should be destroyed; 2) Decides to authorize temporary retention up to not later than 2002 and subject to annual review by the World Health Assembly of the existing stocks of variola virus..."
- It was evident during the smallpox program that a failed eradication effort could have serious repercussions for other global initiatives. Financial support for smallpox eradication was problematic throughout its course, largely because of a failed WHO-sponsored global malaria eradication program after the investment of more than $2 billion. Thus, the credibility of expert public health advice was at a low ebb, and most countries did not want any involvement with another eradication fiasco.
- Sustaining interest and support among countries was extremely difficult, especially after a nil incidence was achieved. Each country was understandably anxious to transfer money and manpower to deal with other critical health problems as soon as possible. They were not enthusiastic about sustaining two or more years of intensive surveillance to confirm that eradication had been achieved. This needs to be borne in mind for eradication campaigns that would need to be phased-in over a long period.

In brief, eradication is not a program to be undertaken lightly. To do so before the necessary technology is clearly in hand and before the practicability of eradication has been demonstrated in the field is an invitation for costly failure and, more importantly, a loss of professional public health and medical credibility.

THE NEXT TARGET AFTER POLIO: GLOBAL ERADICATION OF MEASLES

Stephen L. Cochi, M.D., M.P.H., Peter M. Strebel, M.D., Mark Papania, William J. Bellini, Walter A. Orenstein, M.D.*

*Director, Vaccine-Preventable Disease Eradication Division
National Immunization Program
Centers for Disease Control and Prevention, Atlanta, GA

Despite the availability of highly effective measles vaccines, measles results in approximately 900,000 deaths each year, half of which occur in Africa. The complications of measles (such as bronchopneumonia, diarrhea, and blindness) are most severe in malnourished young children, especially those with vitamin A deficiency. Based on estimates by WHO, each year measles accounts for 30% of all deaths due to vaccine-preventable diseases and 7% of deaths due to all causes among children under five years of age. In 1995, an estimated \$1.1 billion was spent worldwide on measles treatment.

In 1997, the Dahlem Conference on Disease Eradication established three fundamental criteria to be met before a disease is considered eradicable:

1) humans must be critical to maintaining circulation of the organism,
2) sensitive and specific diagnostic tools must be available, and
3) an effective intervention must be available.

Additionally, many experts have established a fourth criterion: demonstration of interruption of transmission for a prolonged period in a large geographic area. Measles meets all four criteria in several ways.

Humans Critical for Transmission

Humans are critical to the maintenance of measles virus transmission; humans are the only reservoir for measles virus, and virus survival in the environment is limited to several hours. The major cell receptor for measles virus, CD46, is found only in primate cells (and in transgenic laboratory animals).

Measles infections have been documented in non-human primates, and epizootics of measles among monkeys can occur in captive colonies in research facilities. However, serological evidence of infection is uncommon among non-human primates in limited contact with humans. Mathematical models and measles epidemiology studies in island populations have estimated that sustained transmission of measles requires a threshold population of at least several hundred thousand. Non-human primate communities do not have sufficient population size or inter-community mixing to sustain measles virus transmission.

Sensitive and Specific Diagnostic Tools

The clinical diagnosis of measles may be useful when measles is common but is unreliable when measles is rare. Thus, greater reliance on laboratory diagnosis based on serologic and salivary assays becomes increasingly important as fewer cases are reported. Capture ELISA tests for IgM on serum have been developed at CDC and are considered the reference standard in the Americas. Using nucleoprotein antigen grown in baculoviruses, these tests have been ≥95% specific and at least 90% sensitive. Approximately 77% of confirmed measles cases are positive by 72 hours and 100% between 72 hours and 11 days following rash onset. Ninety percent are still positive at 28 days. Commercial kits with similar sensitivity and specificity are available and easier to perform than the CDC assay. In the United Kingdom, enzyme immunoassays are being used on oral fluid specimens. Thus, accurate diagnostic tests are available to meet this criterion for measles eradication.

The serological tests are complemented by virus isolation (using B95A marmoset lymphocyte cells), primarily as a way of tracing chains of transmission. They can be used to determine whether isolated cases or new outbreaks represent indigenous transmission from an existing focus or spread from an international importation. Sequencing of the nucleoprotein gene has led to the delineation of at least 15 genotypes, many of which can be traced and appear to circulate in specific geographic areas.

Effective Intervention

Herd Immunity Threshold

Levels of protection induced by a single dose of vaccine are adequate to interrupt transmission. Mathematical modelers have extended this observation and calculated an age-dependent herd immunity threshold which must be exceeded to interrupt transmission. The younger the average age at infection, the more contagious the disease and the higher the immunity level needed. While herd immunity is a mathematical concept and cannot be relied upon to be an absolute predictor as to whether transmission will or will not occur in a specific instance, it provides a target for measles eradication programs.

Based on calculations (Anderson and May, 1992; Hethcote, 1983), the herd immunity threshold in the United States and Europe is at least 93–95%. Levels needed in developing countries may be higher, particularly in urban areas, because the average age at infection may be lower. Generally, however, a target of approximately 95% population immunity seems reasonable.

Failure to Prevent Transmission with a Single Dose

Based on seroconversion and clinical effectiveness studies, a single dose of measles vaccine administered in the second year of life induces immunity in about 95% of vaccinees. In the developing world, persistent transmission of measles virus and high infant morbidity and mortality have led to the recommendation that infants be vaccinated at nine months of age, even though maternal antibody may interfere with seroconversion. Seroconversion rates at nine months of age average 85%. This reduction in seroconversion may seem slight, but a seroconversion rate of 85% leaves three times more infants susceptible (i.e., 15% of vaccinees) than does a rate of 95% (i.e., 5% of vaccinees). Thus, this policy sacrifices maximum seroconversion in an attempt to protect infants at a younger age. A single dose is clearly inadequate to reach a 95% immunity level.

However, if a second dose is given in the second year of life, immunity levels can be increased substantially; at 85% coverage for two independent doses, immunity levels reach 95%. Indeed, all countries attempting to eliminate measles transmission have used some form of two-dose strategy.

Demonstration of Prolonged Interruption

In recent years, major successes in measles elimination—the interruption of indigenous measles transmission but with continued vaccination activities due to the threat of imported cases—from large geographic areas suggest that global eradication is feasible.

Because of its potential for eradication and because global eradication efforts would protect against measles importation, the United States has made measles a global health priority. It has been estimated that the United States would save $45 million or more annually if measles were eradicated and vaccination stopped.

In 1990, the United States supported the World Summit for Children goal to vaccinate 90% of the world's infants with the six EPI (Expanded Program on Immunization) antigens (measles, mumps, rubella, diphtheria, pertussis, tetanus) by 2000. Also in 1990, the United States reaffirmed the World Health Assembly goals of measles morbidity and mortality reduction of 90% and 95%, respectively, compared with pre-vaccine era levels. In 1994, the United States supported the Pan American Health Organization (PAHO) initiative to eliminate measles from the Western Hemisphere by 2000. Similar elimination goals have been adopted by the European region (by 2007) and the eastern Mediterranean region (by 2010).

Four complementary strategies are being used to achieve either measles control or elimination:

- Vaccination (routine and/or supplemental)
- Vitamin A supplementation
- Case management
- Surveillance

The difference between control and elimination strategies is the intensity with which vaccination and surveillance activities are implemented

TABLE 2-1 Measles Control versus Elimination strategies

	Control	Elimination
Routine Immunization	1 dose ≥ 90% coverage	2 doses ≥ 95% coverage
Supplementary Immunization	High-risk areas 9 months to 5 years	Nationwide Broad age range
Surveillance	Integrate with AFP Aggregate case counts	Virus isolation Case-based Lab confirmation

(Table 2-1). Greater than 90% coverage with one dose of vaccine is the recommended WHO policy for achieving measles control. Elimination activities require higher coverage (≥95% in each district or county) with both the first and second doses, whether administered routinely or through nationwide campaigns. Disease surveillance for elimination requires a change from aggregate district level reporting to investigating all suspected measles cases (using serological testing and virus isolation). Genomic sequencing of virus isolates can then help to distinguish indigenous from imported strains.

Figure 2-1 shows reported worldwide number of measles cases and routine vaccination coverage among 1-year-old children. The number of reported measles cases decreased from approximately 4 million in 1983 to 800,000 cases in 1994 and has stayed at that level for the past several years. Routine coverage (black line in the graph) increased during the 1980s to reach 80% in 1990, but has shown no further increase since that time. During the 1990s, there was a substantial decrease in international donor funding for immunization services in developing countries. However, because measles reporting is incomplete, the actual burden from measles in 1996 is an estimated 36.5 million cases and 1 million deaths (Murray and Lopez, 1996). There is optimism that the newly formed Global Alliance for Vaccines and Immunization will increase funding for measles vaccination coverage.

Supplemental measles vaccination campaigns are increasingly being used to supplement routine immunization services and eliminate the build-up of susceptible populations. Nationwide "catch-up" and "follow-up" campaigns are being conducted in an effort to interrupt measles virus transmission. High-risk area campaigns are being conducted to reduce measles cases and deaths in the short term. As of 1998, there has been a 72% reduction in measles cases and an 84% reduction in deaths since the prevaccine era. However, the target goals of global reduction in measles morbidity and mortality have not been achieved.

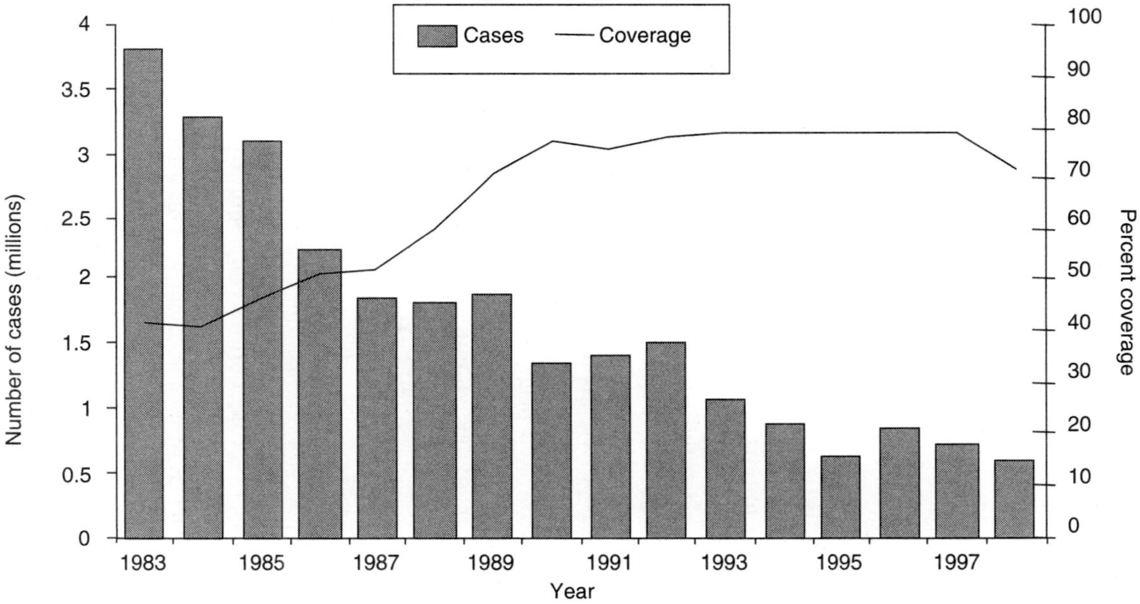

FIGURE 2-1 Reported number of measles cases and routine measles vaccination coverage among 1-year-old children, by year—worldwide, 1983–1998. NOTE: Reported to WHO headquarters, as of August 8, 1999. SOURCE: CDC.

The impacts of routine vaccination and catch-up and follow-up campaigns on the number of reported measles cases in the Americas are shown in Figure 2-2. In 1990, approximately 250,000 measles cases were reported; this decreased by 99% to just over 2,000 cases in 1996. In 1997, over 50,000 cases were reported as a result of a large outbreak of measles among predominantly unvaccinated young adults in Sao Paulo State, Brazil. By 1998, measles had spread from Brazil to other countries in the hemisphere, but the total number of confirmed cases decreased to approximately 15,000 cases. This declining trend continued in 1999, when 3,018 cases were confirmed, and again in 2001, when only 1,755 measles cases were reported, the lowest number ever reported in the Western Hemisphere. In 2000, the intensive efforts to eliminate measles in the Americas led to interruption of measles transmission in 42 of 47 countries or territories.

During the resurgence of measles in the United States from 1989 to 1991, most imported cases were from Mexico and other Latin American countries. Aggressive efforts to eliminate measles in Central and South America during the early 1990s were associated with a marked decrease in the number of measles importations from these countries. By 1996, no importations from Latin America were detected in the United States. In 1997, five importations occurred from Brazil. In 1998 and 1999, zero and two importations were reported from Latin America countries, respectively. In 2000, there have been no importations.

The African Region reported a routine vaccination coverage of 49% in 1998, when an estimated 500,000 children died from measles. Efforts to accelerate measles control have been conducted since the mid-1990s and include: mass vaccination campaigns usually targeting children between nine months and five years of age; vitamin A supplementation administered on polio National Immunization Days (NIDs); strengthened disease surveillance; and PAHO-style measles elimination activities in six southern African countries.

The annual number of reported measles cases in six southern African countries from 1987 to 1999, during which time these countries experienced a rapidly expanding HIV epidemic, is shown in Figure 2-3. Nationwide catch-up campaigns, targeting children nine months to fifteen years of age, conducted from 1996 to 1998, resulted in a >95% reduction in reported cases and the absence of measles deaths. This success demonstrates that despite very high HIV seroprevalence, measles can be well controlled and possibly eliminated.

Recommendations from a Technical Working Group

Recommendations from a Technical Working Group meeting held at WHO in May 2000 will lead to important changes in global measles con-

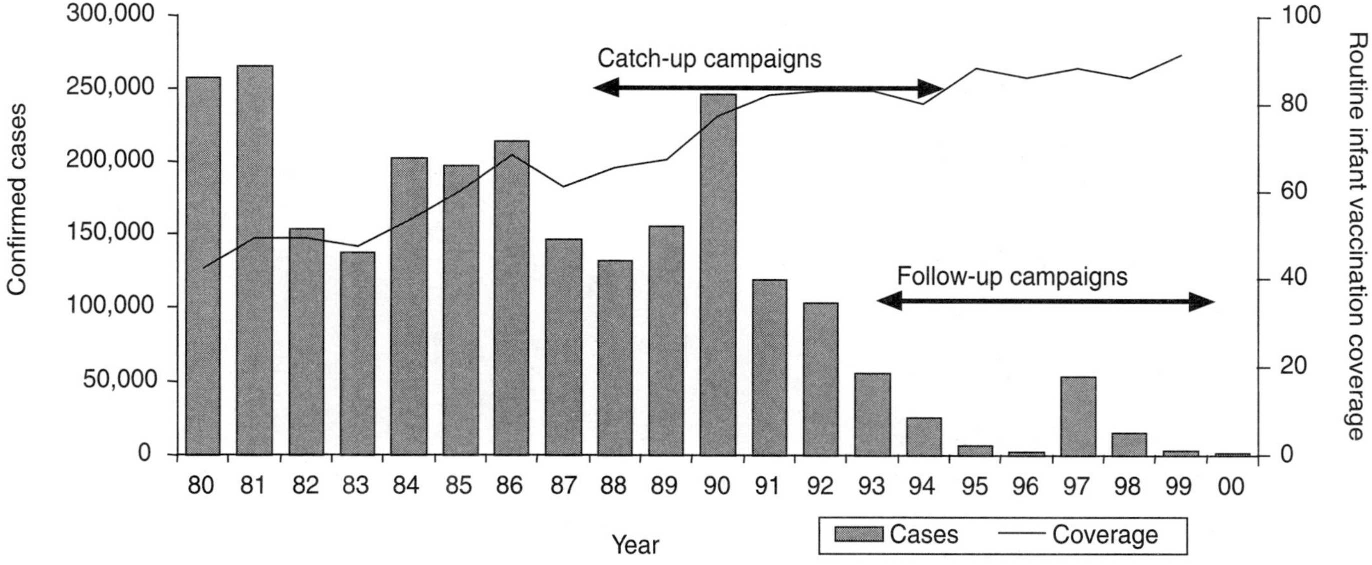

FIGURE 2-2 Vaccination coverage and reported number of measles cases, Region of the Americas, 1980–2000. Data based on 1,564 confirmed cases as of December 20, 2000.
SOURCE: PAHO/WHO.

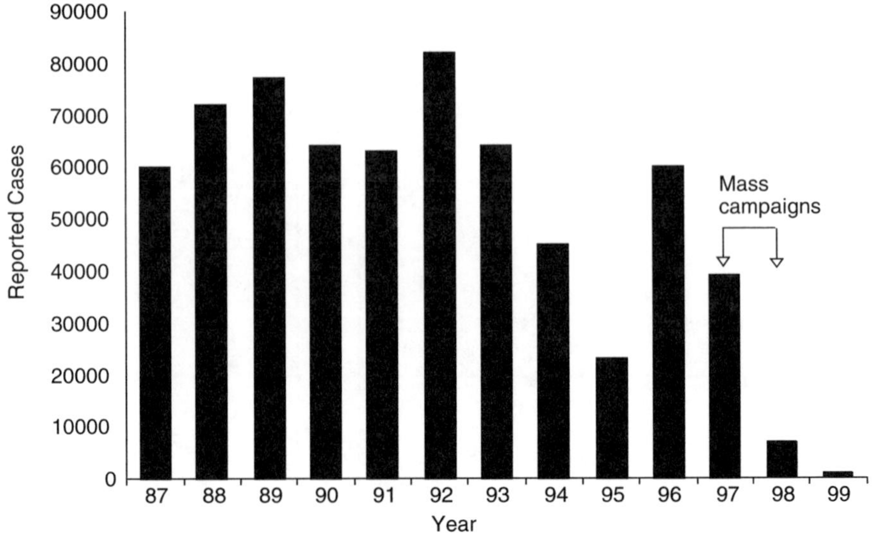

FIGURE 2-3 Reported measles cases in southern Africa during a rapidly expanding HIV epidemic, 1987–1999.

trol. To achieve good measles control, it is now recommended that a one-dose policy is not enough; a second opportunity for measles vaccination should be provided to all children. This can be done through regular mass campaigns or through addition of a routine second dose.

Vaccination campaigns targeting urban communities have only limited impact on measles transmission. In contrast, PAHO-style nationwide campaigns which reach previously unvaccinated children are highly effective at interrupting measles transmission. They should be repeated at regular intervals and integrated with routine immunization services.

Challenges to Global Measles Control and Eradication

Substantial progress has been made toward achieving global measles control and regional elimination goals. However, much remains to be done. The following major challenges need to be met:

1. Interruption of indigenous measles transmission in the Americas by the end of 2001.
2. Implementation of the second opportunity for measles vaccination for all children, and integration of this with the provision of existing immunization services.

3. Development of political and financial support for measles control and a future global eradication initiative.

4. Implementation of special efforts to ensure the safety of injections (both those used during campaigns and those used for routine immunization).

5. Ongoing evaluation of existing strategies, and research and development of new vaccination and surveillance tools.

Impediments to Measles Eradication

There are several impediments to measles eradication:

Transmission among adults

When the measles outbreak in Sao Paulo occurred, it was not clear whether it was only an unusual but transient epidemic caused by high rates of migration of susceptible adults into densely crowded conditions, or if the chain of transmission among adults would persist. Even though it did spread to adults in other countries in Latin America, no other outbreaks were similar in size, suggesting that transmission dies out if adults are the only population capable of transmission.

Increasing urbanization

Densely populated urban centers, even those with a strong immunization program, are ideal settings for prolonged measles transmission. Vaccination programs need to immunize fast enough to prevent accumulation of susceptible children and immigrants, which could fuel outbreaks. Evidence that this is not insurmountable comes from the success of the measles elimination program in Mexico City, the second most populous city in the world. No cases of measles were confirmed in Mexico City in 1998 and 1999. In 2000, 20 measles cases were reported in metropolitan Mexico City. Other major cities with near zero measles incidence include New York, London, and Los Angeles.

However, none of these cities have the population density seen in cities like Bombay, Jakarta, and Lagos, all of which have population densities that are more than three times that of Mexico City. Thus, it remains to be demonstrated whether the immunity levels achieved through the PAHO mass campaigns using existing measles vaccines are capable of eliminating transmission in the population-dense urban areas of Africa and Asia. A critical issue is whether high immunity levels in children nine months to fourteen years of age are sufficient to stop transmission among children younger than nine months of age. If not, there will be a need for vaccines that are more effective in young infants. These concerns have been raised in the past in both the United States and Latin America, but experience has shown that existing measles vaccines in some form of a two-dose schedule are adequate to terminate transmission.

The HIV epidemic

In many areas of the world, particularly in sub-Saharan Africa, up to 30% of women at delivery are infected with HIV. Assuming a 33% rate of maternal-to-infant transmission, an estimated 10% of infants will become infected with HIV.

HIV can cause problems for measles eradication in at least two important ways. First, measles vaccine immunogenicity and presumed effectiveness is substantially lower in HIV-infected persons than in the general population. Nevertheless, data from South Africa, where HIV seroprevalence is 22% among pregnant women (in 1999), show that measles can be markedly reduced and transmission probably terminated even in places with high HIV prevalence. Second, there is the theoretical risk that HIV-infected persons could become chronic measles carriers, transmitting the measles virus years after infection. Further research is needed to address this issue.

Political will

Probably the greatest impediment to eradication is political will, particularly in the developed world where measles may not be seen as a problem. Table 2-2 shows that some of the lowest measles vaccine coverage rates are in some of the world's richest countries. Malawi, with a Gross National Product (GNP) of $170 per capita, reported an 89% coverage rate in 1998. In contrast, Japan, with a GNP of $39,640, reported a coverage rate of only 69%. Measles eradication will require that the developed world realize that measles disease is worth preventing in their own countries so that they do not become reservoirs of the virus. Further, successful eradication will require the developed world to help finance developing country efforts. In the developing world, health authorities will need to be confident that embarking on measles eradication will not detract from delivery of other health services and will lead to benefits for overall health care.

Considerations for Future Measles Eradication

If measles eradication occurs in the future, a number of considerations would need to be addressed before measles vaccination can be stopped in the post-eradication era:

TABLE 2-2 Per Capita Gross National Product (GNP) and Measles Vaccination Coverage

Country	GNP ($US)	Percent Coverage
Malawi	170	89
Vietnam	240	93
Tajikistan	340	80
China	620	97
Italy	19,020	50
Austria	26,890	60
Germany	27,510	75
Japan	39,640	69

SOURCE: UNICEF Data 1998.

- The possibility of long-term excretion of measles virus in HIV-infected, malnourished, or other children will need to be explored and studied.
- The measles virus and potentially infectious materials would need to be contained in the laboratory (based on how the poliovirus was biocontained).
- The possibility of as yet undetected animal reservoirs will need to be explored. The strategy to stop measles vaccination will require wide review and consultation on the possibility of a persistent human or animal reservoir and its implications.
- Given the very high contagiousness and morbidity of measles, this virus represents a substantially higher level of bioterrorist threat than poliovirus, raising concerns among some as to the advisability of discontinuing measles vaccination.

Economic analyses of the benefits of terminating vaccinations should be carefully weighed with all of the above considerations. An alternative to terminating vaccination may be to drop from the existing two-dose measles vaccine schedule to a one-dose schedule.

There are reasons to be optimistic about the prospects for measles eradication. Data from the Americas show that measles transmission can be interrupted, at least transiently, in entire continents. Countries in other regions are now documenting similar success. The available information supports the technical feasibility of measles eradication. Although much work remains to be done to strengthen surveillance and ensure full implementation of the PAHO measles elimination strategy in all countries, there is optimism that the goal of eliminating measles from the Western Hemisphere by the end of 2001 or shortly thereafter will be reached. However, as with all eradication programs, much is learned during implementation, and we must be prepared to modify strategies as experience is gained.

In summary, the world is not yet ready for a global measles eradication initiative. Polio eradication must be achieved first. Nevertheless, the available scientific and programmatic information is encouraging, and we believe someday there will be a goal of measles eradication. Meanwhile, the regional efforts to eliminate measles should be supported, and research should be encouraged to address the potential impediments to global eradication of measles.

ERADICATION OF CONGENITAL RUBELLA SYNDROME

Stanley A. Plotkin, M.D.

Medical and Scientific Consultant, Aventis Pasteur, Swiftwater, PA

Although recognized since the 18th century, rubella was considered a rather benign childhood disease until, during the early days of the Second World War, Australian ophthalmologist Norman McAlister Gregg noticed that most infants with congenital cataracts were born to mothers who shared a maternal history of rubella during early pregnancy. This was the first documented report of congenital rubella syndrome (CRS), a serious disease resulting from infection of the fetus with the rubella virus.

Despite Gregg's earlier observations, the virulence of rubella virus for the fetus was not fully appreciated until the early 1960s, when a rubella pandemic involving millions of cases of infection swept through Europe and the United States. An estimated 20,000 infants were born with CRS, and an estimated 5,000 therapeutic abortions were performed. Even years later, victims of the 1960s pandemic were still recognizable from their CRS sequelae, which include blindness, deafness, and mental retardation. This tragedy confirmed that rubella during the first trimester of pregnancy carries with it a very high risk of fetal damage that warranted prophylaxis.

Pathogenesis and Epidemiology

The rubella virus is a respiratory pathogen which is transmitted either through contact with respiratory secretions of an infected person (i.e., from nasopharynx to nasopharynx), or, in pregnant women, transplacentally to the fetus. Fetal infection may produce spontaneous abortion, stillbirth, CRS, or, occasionally, normal infants. In the case of CRS, the damaging mechanisms—mitotic inhibition and apoptosis—lead to the destruction of the ocular lens, growth retardation, bone lesions, and general derangement of organ development in the fetus. The virus also damages the vascular endothelium, which is probably the cause of encephalitis, central nervous system problems, and damage to the cochlea. Some defects may not become manifest until later in life.

The greatest risk of CRS occurs in the first trimester. Studies in the United Kingdom and the United States show that infection during the first eight weeks of gestation results in 50–90% abnormal fetuses. If infection occurs during the next four to eight weeks, this figure drops to about 33.3%. After about seventeen weeks, there is little evidence of damage. Clinical effects include central nervous system and vision problems, deafness, congenital cardiac disease—particularly PDA (patent ductus arteriosus) and peripheral pulmonic stenosis—and other nonspecific effects.

Rubella epidemiology follows three general patterns:

- In developed countries, pre-vaccination peak age of infection is around school age. Prevalence of seronegative women is 5–20%.
- In island populations, pre-vaccination peak age depends on how recently rubella had been introduced. Prevalence of seronegative women is 20–50%.
- In developing countries, the peak age of infection is pre-school age, and the prevalence of seronegative women is sometimes less than 5%. However, many countries and regions of large countries show much higher prevalence of seronegativity (Cutts et al., 1997).

Diagnosis

Accurate diagnosis of both acquired rubella and CRS has important implications for surveillance issues and documentation of eradication or control. The most sensitive diagnostic technique is reverse transcriptase PCR, which can be used to detect either acquired rubella or CRS by identifying the presence of the virus in nasopharyngeal swabs, blood, or urine. However, PCR is not well adapted to field use. IgM antibody testing is more suited to use in the field. The IgM antibody is generally present for one to two months in acquired rubella and six to twelve months in CRS and can be used to detect either acquired rubella or CRS. Avidity determinations on IgG antibody is another useful diagnostic tool but it can only be performed in sophisticated laboratories and it is not well suited to public health uses. Thus, the most sensitive diagnostic techniques are not suited to or available for field use, and diagnoses often rely on clinical criteria.

The major clinical criteria of CRS are cataracts, glaucoma, retinopathy, heart disease, and central deafness. Minor criteria include purpura, hepatosplenomegaly, microcephaly, developmental delay, meningoencephalitis, and radiolucent bone lesions. As with the criteria for rheumatic fever, the presence of two major criteria is a very likely diagnosis of CRS because there are not very many other congenital problems that cause the same set of signs. The presence of one major and one minor criterion also mean a likely CRS diagnosis.

Cataracts are the simplest clinical finding to detect in the field. Cataracts are present in an estimated 25–35% of all CRS cases, and in the developing world an estimated 25% of all cataracts are due to CRS. If cataracts can be clinically detected in infants, then a very rough estimate of the number of CRS cases in an area can be calculated by multiplying the number of infants with confirmed rubella by four.

Prevention Efforts

Prevention efforts in developed nations rely on the attenuated rubella vaccine, which was developed over 30 years ago. The seroconversion rate is routinely above 95%, and the resistance to reinfection considerable. In one study (Best et al., 1987), 70% of seronegatives challenged with rubella virus developed viremia, and 100% developed viral excretion; 0% of seropositive and vaccinated individuals developed viremia, and 5% of seropositive and vaccinated individuals developed viral excretion. Other studies suggest that naturally seropositive and vaccinated individuals show 95% protection against rubella when clinical criteria are applied and nearly 100% protection when confirmed by laboratory diagnosis. Other data show that even though re-infection following either natural disease or vaccination is a true phenomenon, it does not appear to play a significant role in the epidemiology of this disease.

The primary safety issue concerning the vaccine—a topic relevant to eradication attempts—is possible transmission of live virus to the fetus from either intentional or inadvertent vaccination during pregnancy, or more often, vaccination during inadvertent pregnancy. However, transmission to the fetus rarely occurs, and no CRS defects have been observed in infants born to women vaccinated during early pregnancy (CDC, 1989; Enders, 1984; Tookey et al., 1991). Thus, the safety margin for the rubella vaccine is wide, even though transmission to the fetus during pregnancy remains a contraindication.

The application of vaccination has been fairly complete throughout the Americas and in Scandinavia (Pebody et al., 2000). The United States reported only 567 cases from 1994–1997, 85% of which were in unvaccinated individuals 15 years of age or older (CDC, 1997). Interestingly, 54% of these cases were Latino, reflecting the non-use of rubella vaccine in Latin America. Recently, however, the situation has begun to change. There seems to be interruption of indigenous transmission in Mexico due to the introduction of the rubella vaccine there, and an increasing proportion of imported cases in the United States come from Europe, Japan, and elsewhere. According to WHO, the percentage of countries in the Americas using the vaccine has been approaching 50%, and by now that percentage has probably reached 100%.

Thus far, the best rubella control has been achieved in Scandinavia, where two doses of vaccine have been systematically administered since the early 1980s. In continental Europe, however, the disease has far from disappeared because of considerable resistance to the use of rubella and measles vaccines. For example, the United Kingdom's control efforts are in danger because of rumors linking measles vaccination to autism (DeStefano and Chen, 1999).

The situation in the rest of the world is mixed. Immunization rates are increasing in the eastern Mediterranean, Southeast Asia, and western Pacific regions. However, the world's two most populous countries, India and China, do not use rubella vaccine routinely, nor do Africa and large parts of Asia.

Currently, there are an estimated 100 CRS cases per 100,000 live births in countries where the rubella vaccine is not used, which amounts to approximately 100,000 CRS cases per year worldwide (see Table 2-3). Although rubella mortality is not as high as that of measles, the large number of CRS cases signifies a large population of handicapped individuals. There does not appear to be any geographical variation in the virulence of rubella virus for the fetus.

Recent situations in Vellore, India, and Kumasi, Ghana, exemplify the widespread nature of the disease. In Vellore, India, over 200 cases of CRS were detected over a four-year period in a hospital with 10,000 annual births, yielding a rate of about five per 1,000 live births. Because these cases were diagnosed on the basis of clinical criteria and not confirmed with laboratory assays, this figure may be an overestimate. Nevertheless, even if the true figure were only a portion of this, it would still be high. In Kumasi, Ghana, there was an epidemic—30,000 reported cases—of rash disease in 1995 (Lawn et al., 2000). Local investigators used IgM assays to detect 18 cases of CRS, suggesting a *minimum* incidence of 0.8 per 1,000 live births. Assuming that rubella immunity was 92.5%, the investigators estimated that 3,000 pregnant women were infected with rubella and 700 babies born with CRS during the epidemic.

Eradication of Rubella

There are several reasons to be optimistic about the eradication of rubella and/or CRS. First, there is no animal reservoir (one of the preconditions for eradication, as discussed in Chapter 1). Second, human reservoirs

TABLE 2-3 Mean Estimated Incidence Rate of CRS per 100,000 Live Births and Number of Cases of CRS by WHO Region, 1996 (Cutts and Vynnycky, 1999)

WHO Region	Incidence rate of CRS per 100,000 live births	Number of CRS cases
Africa	104	22,471
Americas		
Island	171	
Mainland	175	
Total		15,994
Eastern Mediterranean	77	12,080
Southeast Asia	136	46,621
Western Pacific	173	12,634
Global Total		109,800

are transitory and probably not very important at the public health level. Even though congenitally infected infants do excrete the virus, they stop excreting it when they acquire cellular, particularly CD4-mediated, immunity. Although there are rare cases of encephalitis in which virus persists in the brain, there have been no reported cases of excretion. And, so far, there is no example of an immunosuppressed individual continuing to excrete. Third, the rubella vaccine is effective and available in combination with the measles vaccine. The latter is significant because a measles-rubella (MR) or a measles-mumps-rubella (MMR) vaccine would not increase administration costs in places where these other vaccines are currently available.

Thus, CRS eradication by correct application of measles-rubella-containing vaccines is feasible. Nonetheless, potential eradication efforts face several challenges:

- Although the administration cost would be the same, adding the mumps and/or rubella components to the measles vaccine would increase the price of the vaccine to approximately 30 to 50 cents per dose.
- Vaccine supply needs to meet demand, which would require encouraging manufacturers to increase production, and also would lead to price reduction.
- Decreasing the circulation of rubella among children may leave women who grow up without contact with the virus more susceptible to infection, thereby increasing their risk of acquired rubella and paradoxically increasing the number of CRS cases in parts of the world where, ordinarily, women grow up immune.

- Unlike measles where a rash is an almost uniform manifestation of infection, rubella infections can be completely subclinical or without a rash.

Eradication strategies differ between the developed and developing world. In developed countries, the current strategy—universal MMR at 12 to 18 months and again at 4 to 12 years, plus vaccination of adolescents and adults at any opportunity—is successful and should continue. In developing countries, rubella should be added to the measles vaccine, and universal immunization with combination MR vaccines at 9 to 12 months of age should be increased. Also in order to avoid paradoxical increases in CRS in developing countries, repeated, mass vaccination campaigns should be directed at children between 1 and 14 years of age in order to interrupt circulation of the virus. Attempts to vaccinate older individuals may be complicated by the lack of health service infrastructure and experience, as well as increased risk of reactogenicity and contraindication for use in adult women.

In conclusion, CRS can be readily controlled. It could even be eradicated or eliminated in adult women by the correct application of combination MR vaccines. However, because of the challenges that inapparent infections create, neither eradication of the virus nor post-eradication discontinuation of vaccination is foreseeable in the near future.

POST-POLIO ERADICATION: ISSUES AND CHALLENGES

Walter R. Dowdle, Ph.D.

Public Health Consultant, Task Force for Child Survival and Development, Atlanta, GA

In the late 1950s, Albert Sabin, Hilary Kaproski, and others concluded that routine immunization (with either inactivated polio vaccine [IPV] or oral live-attenuated polio vaccine [OPV]), which had proven so successful at interrupting poliovirus transmission in developed countries, would not be effective in high-risk developing countries where social and environmental conditions favor continuous virus transmission. Instead, Sabin proposed mass OPV immunization, which has proven to be the most effective strategy for the control of poliomyelitis epidemics in the developing world (Sabin, 1985). Global eradication is the natural outcome.

Eradication Strategy

The global polio eradication initiative, which is driven by both public and private partnerships and spearheaded by WHO, Rotary International,

CDC, and the United Nations Children's Fund (UNICEF), relies on age-specific routine childhood immunizations supplemented with mass OPV immunization. National immunization days (NIDs) with OPV are conducted two or more times annually for all children under the age of five years. As nationwide polio cases decline, immunization strategies are increasingly targeted to virus reservoir and high-risk population areas through sub-national immunization days and house-to-house mop-up operations.

Aggressive surveillance is key to a successful immunization strategy. All cases of acute flaccid paralysis (AFP) in the country should be reported and investigated, and stool specimens collected for testing in accredited WHO laboratories within two weeks of onset, regardless of clinical diagnosis (Hull et al., 1994). Polioviruses can then be isolated, identified, differentiated as to wild or recent vaccine in origin, and sequenced for genome characterization.

Current Progress

At the time of the 1988 World Health Assembly resolution (WHA, 1988), paralytic polio was endemic in 125 countries on five continents, with an estimated 350,000 cases annually. The last indigenous case in the Americas was in 1991, the Western Pacific Region in 1997, and the European Region in 1998. Wild poliovirus type 2 has not been found anywhere in the world since mid-1999.

In 2000, polio still occurred in 20 countries, with less than 3,000 cases identified worldwide. Slightly more than 250 cases were detected in India, the world's major exporter of wild polioviruses, despite major advances in surveillance. Still, this was down nearly a factor of 10 from the number of cases reported in 1998. Much work remains to be done to mop up poliovirus types 1 and 3 in the Middle East and southeast Asia and Africa, especially in areas of civil conflict and in countries with weak or non-existent health infrastructure. The goal of eradication by 2000 was not met, but the original goal of certifying the world as polio-free by 2005 may still be within reach.

Post-Eradication Strategies

A major reason for polio eradication is that, as with the eradication of smallpox, immunization would no longer be required. However, stopping OPV immunization is no simple matter. The resulting rapid increase in non-immune persons in much of the post-eradication developing world raises concerns that polio could re-emerge from independently circulating OPV-derived viruses, unrecognized natural poliovirus reservoirs, or unintentional or intentional laboratory transmission (Fine and Carneiro, 1998).

In 1997, a WHO technical consultative group recommended that OPV immunization should stop and IPV immunization may stop when there is sufficient assurance that wild polioviruses have been eradicated, vaccine-derived polioviruses are no longer circulating, and the remaining stocks of wild polioviruses and infectious materials have been suitably contained in the laboratory (Wood et al., 2000). Each of these three criteria is addressed below.

Assurance of eradication

The world will be certified polio-free when the Global Commission for the Certification of Polio Eradication is satisfied that all six Regional Commissions and their national committees have provided adequate data to document the absence of wild poliovirus transmission after at least three years of high-quality post-eradication surveillance (WHA, 1988).

Assurance of the absence of circulating OPV-derived wild virus

Sabin OPV strains are genetically unstable and regain certain wild virus characteristics upon replication in the human gut. But high levels of immunity in adequately immunized populations limit opportunities for independent OPV virus circulation. However, inadequately immunized populations represent a considerable risk. Polio caused by independently circulating OPV-derived type 2 viruses is reported to have occurred in the past (CDC, 2001). Recent cases of polio from the island of Hispaniola extend these findings to OPV type 1 as well (CDC, 2000). Adding to the complexity of assuring absence of circulating OPV are the rare immuno-compromised individuals who may shed OPV-derived viruses for a prolonged period of time. Nearly a dozen such persons have been identified worldwide over the last 38 years (Wood et al., 2000). Some have stopped spontaneously; others have shed vaccine-derived poliovirus for up to 10 years or more.

Assurance that laboratory stocks and infectious materials are adequately contained

Absolute containment cannot be assured. Questions of intentional or unintentional non-compliance will always remain. However, effective containment is a realistic goal. To achieve effective containment, the reasons must be clear and compelling, the biosafety requirements appropriate, and the goals realistic.

In theory, inadvertent transmission of viruses from the laboratory to the community may occur through contaminated clothing, liquid or air effluents, or improper disposal of infectious materials. No evidence exists for poliovirus transmission by these routes, but such possibilities are effectively addressed by the appropriate WHO standards for laboratory design and biosafety practices (WHO, 1999). The major challenge presented by poliovirus is to prevent transmission to the community through an unrecognized infectious laboratory worker. For such transmission to occur, four conditions must be met: (1) poliovirus materials must be present in the laboratory, (2) some operation must be performed with those materials that exposes the worker to the virus, (3) the worker must be susceptible to an infection that results in poliovirus shedding and the exposure of others, and (4) those exposed in the community must be susceptible to infection. Blocking transmission by eliminating the first three conditions is currently not possible. But the risks from each of the three conditions can be greatly reduced, collectively providing a high level of community protection and greatly reducing the chances of inadvertent transmission. Reducing the risks of the fourth condition requires alignment of biosafety recommendations with post-eradication immunization policies adopted by the international community.

In December 1999, WHO published the *WHO Global Action Plan for Laboratory Containment of Wild Polioviruses* (WHO, 1999; WHO, 2000). The first step in this widely reviewed plan requires that each nation survey all laboratories that may possess wild poliovirus infectious or potentially infectious materials, encourage the disposition of unneeded materials, and prepare a national inventory of all laboratories that retain such materials.

By the end of the second year after detection of the last wild poliovirus, all laboratories that retain wild poliovirus infectious material will be required to dispose of such materials or institute biosafety level 3 (high containment). Laboratories with potentially infectious materials will be required to implement biosafety procedures appropriate for the risks. Decisions about if, how, and when to stop immunization will directly affect the final containment requirements. If OPV immunization is stopped, the requirement will increase to maximum containment (BSL-4) for wild polioviruses and high containment for all OPV-derived viruses.

Post-Eradication OPV Options

Three post-eradication immunization options may be considered: (1) continue OPV, (2) discontinue OPV after synchronized global immunization days (GIDs), or (3) replace OPV with routine IPV for an indefinite period of time. New OPV strains, even if scientifically possible, are a questionable option because of length of time, costs for development, and practical and ethical considerations that preclude complete field trials in a fully immunized population. Further, genetic stability and rare adverse events would not be known until the vaccine is in widespread use.

Option 1, continuing mass OPV immunization, maintains the status quo and reduces concerns of re-emerging wild virus. The major disadvantage of this strategy is that vaccine-associated paralytic poliovirus (VAPP) continues in developing countries that have neither the health infrastructure nor the funds to convert to IPV. Paradoxically, continuing OPV to avoid the risk of independently circulating OPV-derived viruses is also an argument for stopping it. Maintaining adequate vaccine coverage levels will not be easy in the absence of wild poliovirus, during a time of changing public perception of OPV risk/benefits, and in an era of decreased international funding.

Option 2, stopping OPV after synchronized global immunization days, is based on the observations in Cuba and elsewhere that circulation of OPV strains ceases in a well-immunized population about three months after the last NID (PAHO, 1985). The advantages of this option are the elimination of VAPP and vaccine costs. The disadvantages are the inequities of continuing IPV use in developed countries and absence of any protection in developing countries where the risks of polio re-emergence are greatest. Finally, the unknowns inherent in this option necessitate establishing large OPV stockpiles and rapid response contingency plans, in themselves also unknowns.

Option 3, replacing OPV with IPV, is an attractive option on the surface. Virtually all polio risks are eliminated for the vaccine recipient, IPV can replace OPV on a systematic country-by-country basis, and, most importantly, it can strengthen routine expanded program of immunization (EPI) coverage through combination IPV/DPT (diphtheria-pertussis-tetanus) vaccines. However, the effectiveness of IPV in preventing OPV-derived virus circulation in developing tropical countries is unknown. Finally, the global costs of IPV and demand on production capacity are not fully appreciated.

Conclusion

A world without polio brings with it unprecedented public health challenges and the urgent need for clarity of perspective on appropriate post-eradication actions. With continued high quality surveillance, over time, the absence of circulating wild virus can be assured. With the full commitment of all nations, effective laboratory containment is a realistic goal. However, the potential of OPV-derived polioviruses to establish and maintain circulation in inadequately immunized populations has important post-eradication implications. Decisions about if, how, and when to stop OPV immunization must be based on scientific evidence from continued epidemiological and virological surveillance, poliovirus studies, laboratory containment progress, and further research on post-eradication options. Time is of the essence. OPV acceptance may wane in the absence of wild poliovirus circulation. Of particular urgency is research on the role of IPV and possible combinations of options leading to sound post-eradication strategies.

REFERENCES

Anderson RM and May RM. 1992. *Infectious Diseases of Humans: Dynamics and Control.* Oxford: University of Oxford Press.

Best JM, Welch JM, Baker DA, and Banatvala JE. 1987. Maternal rubella at St Thomas' Hospital in 1978 and 1986: Support for augmenting the rubella vaccination programme. *Lancet* 2(8550):88–90.

Centers for Disease Control and Prevention. 1989. Rubella vaccination during pregnancy—United States, 1971–1988. *Morbidity and Mortality Weekly Report* 38(17):289–293.

Centers for Disease Control and Prevention. 1997. Rubella and congenital rubella syndrome—United States, 1994–1997. *Morbidity and Mortality Weekly Report* 46(16):350–354.

Centers for Disease Control and Prevention. 2000. Outbreak of poliomyelitis—Dominican Republic and Haiti, 2000. *Morbidity and Mortality Weekly Report* 49:1094, 1103.

Centers for Disease Control and Prevention. 2001. Circulation of a type 2 vaccine derived poliovirus, Egypt, 1982–1993. *Morbidity and Mortality Weekly Report* 50(3):41–42, 51.

Cutts FT and Vynnycky E. 1999. Modelling the incidence of congenital rubella syndrome in developing countries. *International Journal of Epidemiology* 28(6):1176–1184.

Cutts FT, Robertson SE, Diaz-Ortega JL, and Samuel R. 1997. Control of rubella and congenital rubella syndrome (CRS) in developing countries, Part 1: Burden of disease from CRS. *Bulletin of the World Health Organization* 75(1):55–68.

DeStefano F and Chen RT. 1999. Negative association between MMR and autism. *Lancet* 353(9169):1987–1988.

Enders G. 1984. Accidental rubella vaccination in pregnancy. *Deutsche medizinische Wochenschrift* 109(47):1806–1809.

Fenner F, Henderson DA, Arita I, Jezek Z, and Ladnyi ID. 1988. *Smallpox and Its Eradication.* Geneva: World Health Organization.

Fine P and Carneiro L. 1998. Transmissibility and persistence of oral polio vaccine viruses: Implications for the global poliomyelitis eradication initiative. *American Journal of Epidemiology* 150(10):1001–1021.

Hethcote HW. 1983. Measles and rubella in the United States. *American Journal of Epidemiology* 117(1):2–13.

Hull HF, Ward NA, Hull BP, Milstien JB, and de Quadros C. 1994. Paralytic poliomyelitis seasoned strategies, disappearing disease. *Lancet* 343:1331–1337.

Jezek Z and Fenner F. 1988. *Human Monkeypox.* Basel, Switzerland: S Karger.

Lawn JE, Reef S, Baffoe-Bonnie B, Adadevoh S, Caul EO, and Griffin GE. 2000. Unseen blindness, unheard deafness, and unrecorded death and disability: Congenital rubella in Kumasi, Ghana. *American Journal of Public Health* 90(10):1555–1561.

Murray JL and Lopez AD. 1996. The global burden of disease: a comprehensive assessment of mortality and disability from diseases, injuries, and risk factors in 1990 and projected to 2020. Geneva: World Health Organization.

Pan American Health Organization (PAHO). 1985. Director announces campaign to eradicate poliomyelitis from the Americas by 1990. *Bulletin of the Pan American Health Organization* 19:213–215.

Pebody RG, Edmunds WJ, Conyn-van Spaendonck M, Olin P, Berbers G, Rebiere I, Lecoeur H, Crovari P, Davidkin I, Gabutti G, Gerike E, Giordano C, Hesketh L, Plesner AM, Raux M, Rota MC, Salmaso S, Tischer A, Valle M, and Miller E. 2000. The seroepidemiology of rubella in western Europe. *Epidemiology and Infection* 125(2):347–357.

Sabin AB. 1985. Oral poliovirus vaccine: History of its development and use and current challenge to eliminate poliomyelitis from the world. *Journal of Infectious Diseases* 151:420–436.

Tookey PA, Jones G, Miller BH, and Peckham CS. 1991. Rubella vaccination in pregnancy. *Communicable Disease Report (London England: Review)* 1(8):R86–R88.

Wood DJ, Sutter RW, and Dowdle WR. 2000. Stopping poliovirus vaccination after eradication: Issues and challenges. *Bulletin of the World Health Organization* 78:347–357.

World Health Assembly. 1988. *Global Eradication of Poliomyelitis by the Year 2000.* Geneva: World Health Organization.

World Health Organization. 1980. *The Global Eradication of Smallpox:* Final Report of the Global Commission for the Certification of Smallpox Eradication. Geneva: World Health Organization.

World Health Organization. 1999. *Global Action Plan for Laboratory Containment of Wild Polioviruses.* Geneva: World Health Organization.

World Health Organization. 2000. *Guidelines for Implementing the Pre-Eradication Phase of the Global Action Plan for Laboratory Containment of Wild Polioviruses.* Geneva: World Health Organization.

3

Biological Challenges to Post-Eradication

OVERVIEW

All of the viruses currently under consideration for eradication rely on highly effective vaccines and well-defined immunization programs to interrupt transmission. Major biological challenges after eradication include:

- knowing how and when to stop immunization;
- improving vaccine technology and production should a vaccine ever be needed even after the cessation of immunization;
- safely containing viruses in the lab in the post-eradication era; and
- continuing and improving surveillance for the detection of vaccine-associated cases, recrudescence of infection, new zoonotic transmissions, and the emergence of recombinant viral strains.

Overcoming these challenges will require a better understanding of pathogen transmission and viral biology.

For example, vaccine-preventable viruses (e.g., polio and measles) are characterized by boom-and-bust epidemic cycles which exhibit extraordinary non-linear dynamics due to the complex population-level interactions that influence transmission. Mathematical modeling that takes these interactions into account provides a robust scientific framework for predicting the impact of mass vaccination and exploring immunization cessation strategies. It can help us answer questions such as: How extensive must vaccination be to interrupt transmission in a defined population? What age class should mass vaccination target? Are catch-up campaigns effective?

Even after eradication and the cessation of immunization, it may not be desirable to completely eliminate all traces of the infectious agent because of its use in basic scientific and vaccine advancement research, as well as the need for an emergency stockpile in case of recrudescence. Thus, post-eradication strategies must consider safe laboratory containment of the virus to minimize the risks of accidental or intentional re-introduction.

In addition to recrudescence of wild-type virus, other potential post-eradication outbreaks could result from vaccine-associated infections, new recombinant strains of virus (e.g., between circulating HIV and newly introduced SIV), or new zoonotic transmissions (e.g., the existence of a primate reservoir must be taken into account while planning future eradication, and eventually post-eradication, strategies for HIV/AIDS). Most notably, vaccine-associated paralytic poliomyelitis (VAPP) demonstrates how vaccine-associated cases of disease can occur even when disease due to wild-type virus is eliminated. Post-eradication strategies will require continual surveillance, more information about the duration of shedding and the persistence of the vaccine-derived virus in the environment, and continuing vaccine coverage even in areas where wild-type virus has been eradicated.

Viruses have extraordinary evolutionary strategies about which we have very little understanding. Continual surveillance and improved sampling methods are essential for tracking new genetic variants, particularly as more vaccines are introduced worldwide and rarer genotypes are selected for. The chance that new viruses could evolve underscores the need for continued development of improved vaccines and vaccine delivery systems.

HERD IMMUNITY AND THE DESIGN OF VACCINATION PROGRAMS

Professor Roy M. Anderson, Ph.D., F.R.S.

Department of Infectious Disease Epidemiology
Imperial College School of Medicine
University of London, London, U.K.

The past four decades have witnessed remarkable success in the control of viral diseases by mass vaccination. The most notable of these is the eradication of smallpox in 1977 (Fenner et al., 1988), which resulted from an intensive worldwide immunization campaign. The success of the smallpox campaign has provided hope that other viral infections for which effective and safe vaccines are available—particularly polio and measles—can also be eradicated, given the will and financial resources. However, there are still many problems associated with pathogen transmission that must be resolved before eradication can be achieved. These problems result from variation in vaccine uptake among countries, increased mixing of populations between cities and towns worldwide, and the high transmissibility of viruses within high-density populations.

The development of a safe, effective, and cheap vaccine is only the first step—albeit a vital one—toward community-based control of infectious disease. Population-level processes, such as the demography of the human host, human behavior, and the biological factors that influence transmission all play critical roles in determining the impact of mass vaccination. The dynamics of the interaction between an infectious agent and its human host population are complex and often highly non-linear in form due to variation in the course of infection within the human host and the interaction of demography (e.g., net birth rate) and host behavior (e.g., patterns of mixing) (Anderson, 1994). The resultant complex patterns are often seasonal; they are driven by both climatic influences on the likelihood of transmission and changes in behavior (e.g., school attendance and aggregation of children). They can also be longer-term as a result of the dynamic interaction between the exhaustion (by infection) and renewal (by new births) of the supply of susceptible individuals. Longer-term cycles occurred in many developed countries prior to and after the initiation of routine mass immunization and are a well-known phenomenon.

Once mass vaccination is initiated within a defined community, these complex interactions may be influenced in a manner that is not easily understood in the absence of a detailed template for analysis and interpretation. Mathematical models that combine the processes underlying the typical course of infection in the host with those that determine transmission between hosts provide a robust scientific framework for the prediction of intervention impact and the formulation of cost-effective policies (Anderson and May, 1990; Anderson et al., 1997). This summary provides a review of recent progress in this type of mathematical modeling, with a particular focus on the factors that influence the persistence of infection and disease in communities with high rates of vaccine uptake. The childhood vaccine-preventable viral and bacterial infections, such as measles, mumps, rubella, polio, and pertussis, provide the empirical basis for much of the theory.

Basic Principles

Simple theory provides many insights into the likely impact of a defined immunization program targeted at a particular infectious agent. One of the central epidemiological concepts underlying this theory is the basic reproductive number, R_0, which is defined as the average number of secondary cases of infection generated by one primary case in a susceptible community. The magnitude of R_0 is determined by a blend of parameters that influence the typical course of infection within the human host with parameters that determine transmission between individuals. For a directly transmitted viral or bacterial infection that exhibits little antigenic variability (i.e., one dominant serotype), the approximate value of R_0 is given by the expression:

$$R_0 = [L - A]/[A - M],$$

where L is human life expectancy, M is the average duration of protection from maternally derived antibodies, and A is the average age of infection in an unvaccinated community. The value of L can be replaced by an equivalent term representing the net birth rate of the community, since it is this parameter that generates the renewal of the supply of susceptibles. For example, for measles in the United States prior to wide-scale immunization, with L, A, and M values of 70, 5, and 0.5, respectively, each primary case of infection generated 14 to 15 secondary cases in a totally susceptible community.

In the case of endemic persistence within a community, where many have recovered from infection and are immune to re-infection, the effective reproductive number, R, is unity in value: each primary case generates, on average, exactly one secondary case. The effective reproductive number, R, is the average number of secondary cases generated by one primary case in a population that is not entirely susceptible to infection (i.e., the presence of those who are immune due to recovery or immunization). In cases where seasonal factors influence transmission and the transmission dynamics of the virus generates longer-term oscillations in incidence, the magnitude of R will fluctuate above and below unity in value.

The magnitude of R_0 in an unvaccinated community can be determined from either cross-sectional or longitudinal serological surveys which define, by age, what percentage of the population is seropositive for specific antigens of an infectious agent. The rate of increase in seropositivity between two age classes provides a quantitative measure of the age-specific incidence of infection, which is sometimes referred to as the "attack rate" or "force of infection."

A serological approach to epidemiological surveillance is much more accurate than case reports of infection, since the latter tend to vary in reliability depending on the prevailing incidence of infection. Under-reporting is common when an infection is rare, and over-reporting can arise during an epidemic phase in a recurrent epidemic situation. Serology works well for viral infections but is more problematic for bacterial disease, due to the decline over time in detectable antibodies to past infection.

A diagrammatic illustration of a cross-sectional serological survey is

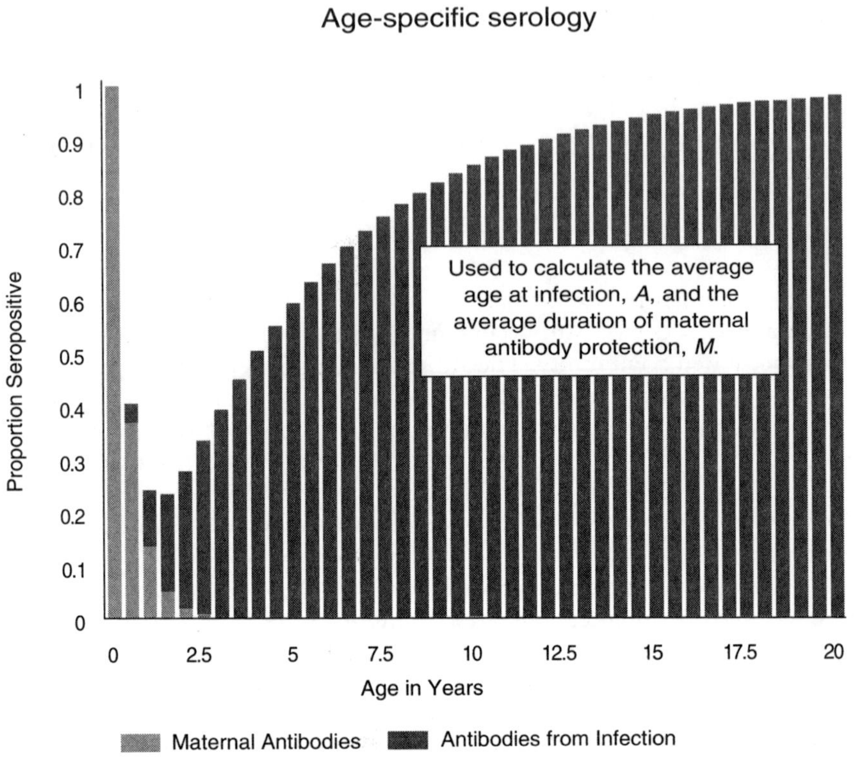

FIGURE 3-1 Diagrammatic example of a cross-sectional serological survey (L = 70 yrs, A = 5 yrs). It records the fraction of a sample of sera collected from a population that are seropositive to the antigens of a defined infectious agent, stratified by host age.

documented in Figure 3-1. The pattern displayed provides considerable information relevant to the design of mass vaccination programs. For example, the trough in susceptibility, which occurs after the decay of maternally derived protection and before the rise resulting from infection, defines the optimum age for vaccination, given the poor efficacy of many vaccines if delivered when the titer of maternally derived antibody is high.

Cross-sectional surveys can be repeated yearly and then combined to provide a longitudinal pattern of immunity and a precise picture of the "herd immunity" profile of a population over time. The specificity and sensitivity of saliva-based serological tests for many viral infections suggest that surveillance based on herd immunity profiles should be more widely adopted. Gaps or troughs in herd immunity profiles can provide policy guidance for the introduction of "top up" age-targeted immunization programs in situations where overall levels of vaccine uptake are moderate to high. If stratified by location and ethnic or other social group, the profiles can also be used to identify social groups or communities with low uptake levels. Finland is exemplary in the quality of serological data collected to monitor infectious disease incidence and the impact of particular mass vaccination programs. Few other countries use this approach to infectious disease surveillance.

Mass Vaccination

Theory also sheds light on the degree of mass immunization required to block transmission in a defined population. If the average age at immunization is *V*, and *A* and *L* are as defined previously, then the critical proportion of each yearly birth cohort that must be effectively immunized to block transmission, p_c, is given by the simple expression (Anderson and May, 1992):

$$p_c = [L - A]/[A - V].$$

The critical fraction is minimized by keeping the value of *V* as low as possible. For infections, such as measles, that have a low average age at infection (*A*), cohort immunization must be very high (typically in excess of 90% to 95%) to block transmission within most urban populations. Theoretically, in rural areas with lower densities and higher average ages at infection, the critical level of uptake to block transmission is somewhat lower. Practically, however, the values of p_c derived for urban areas must be applied even to rural communities due to ever-increasing connectedness between urban and rural areas.

The expression for p_c defined above oversimplifies the tasks required for eradication. For example, two important factors that affect the value of p_c are a decrease in vaccine efficacy in the presence of high titers of maternally derived antibody (these decline rapidly from birth, with a detection half life of roughly 6 months for most viral infections), and vaccines of less than perfect efficacy, even in the absence of maternal antibodies. Both of these factors yield a more complex expression for the value of p_c.

Once p_c is derived, a graph can be plotted for any given infection and vaccine of defined properties relating the average age at vaccination (*V*) and vaccine efficacy (*e*) to the critical fraction of a cohort that must be immunized (p_c) (see Figure 3-2; Anderson et al., 1997). The efficacy of most current vaccines is far less than perfect: estimates range from 72% to 88% for mumps, 90% to 95% for measles, and 96% to 99% for rubella (Plotkin and Orenstein, 1999).

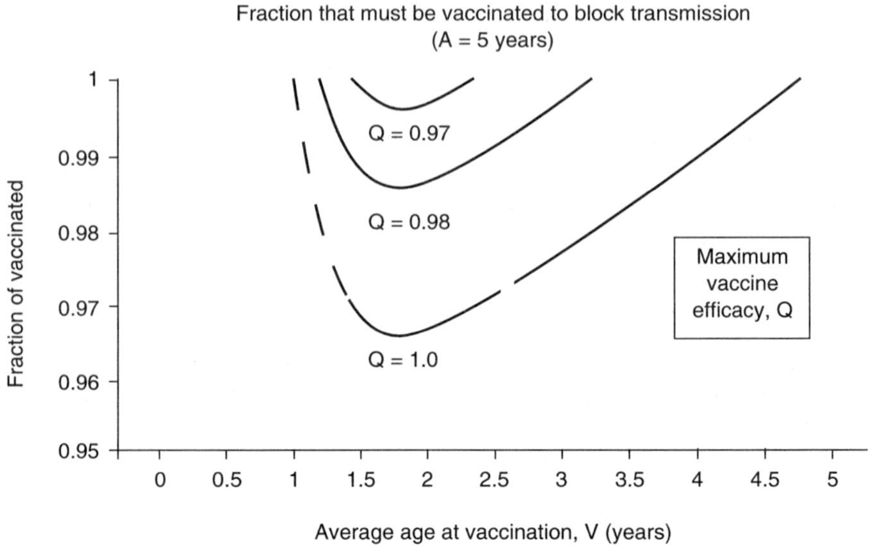

FIGURE 3-2 The impact of age at vaccination and vaccine efficacy on the critical level of cohort vaccination required to block transmission.
NOTE: Vaccine efficacy changes with age due to presence of maternal antibodies.

In the case of highly transmissible infections (high R_0 values), such as measles, a lower than 100% vaccine efficacy strongly hinders the task of blocking transmission. As illustrated in Figure 3-2, the fraction of the cohort that must be immunized in order to block transmission is greater than one, implying that more than one round of immunization of a given cohort is required for effective blockage (i.e., two-stage immunization policies) (Bottiger et al., 1987). Even two-stage immunization may not be sufficient if either the average age at infection is very low, children who are not protected by the first immunization can never be protected due to nutritional or genetic factors, or if those not immunized in the first round of immunization are also not immunized in the second round at a later age. An example of the consequences of low average age at infection is the situation in Lagos, Nigeria, a large city in a developing country with a high birth rate. An average age at infection of around one to two years prior to mass vaccination requires that immunization be effectively administered near birth in order to block transmission. However, if delivered too soon after birth, the presence of maternally derived antibodies significantly reduces vaccine efficacy. In short, the combination of high transmissibility (low average age at infection), imperfect vaccine efficacy, and behavioral or social predisposition to remaining unimmunized suggests that eradication in some parts of the world may be very difficult.

Mass immunization influences the epidemiology of infectious agents in several ways. First, it lowers transmission success (i.e., from infected to still susceptible individuals), thereby increasing the average age at infection. If the likelihood of serious disease resulting from infection increases with age, low to moderate vaccine coverage may increase net morbidity, a particularly worrisome situation for rubella vaccination campaigns in developing countries. Every effort should be made to achieve high uptake. Second, immunization tends to lengthen the inter-epidemic period. Third, a trough of susceptibility moves across the herd immunity profile in older age classes, due to decreased transmission rates and exposure following the mass immunization (see Figure 3-3). All of these epidemiological phenomena, which have been both predicted by theory and observed in practice, need to be considered when monitoring the impact of mass vaccination.

How to Vaccinate and at Which Age

The design of immunization programs involves many different factors, such as cost and sustainability. Developed countries usually use cohort immunization at one or two different ages for any given vaccine or combination of vaccines (e.g., measles-mumps-rubella [MMR]). Practicalities dictate that ease of access to infants and children via health clinics or schools is critical in determining at what age vaccination is offered. It is essential that as high a fraction of children as possible are immunized at as young an age as possible, while taking into account the complexities induced by maternal antibodies. For example, even though many countries offer MMR vaccination at around two years of age, the observed distribution of ages at immunization is not always clustered around this age as it should be.

An alternative or addition to cohort immunization is a pulse or "catch-up" immunization strategy involving particular days (or weeks) designated as "immunization days" and publicized by the press. On immunization days, health care services offer vaccination to all children of a particular age range. Immunization days must occur at regular intervals, perhaps every one to two years in the early stages of the program and less frequently as overall coverage rises and infection incidence falls. This approach has been used with considerable success in South American countries (de Quadros et al., 1996).

Analyses based on mathematical models of viral transmission confirm that catch-up campaigns can effectively disrupt spread, particularly when infections exhibit seasonal oscillatory trends in incidence or inter-epidemic periods lasting a few years (Agur et al., 1993). The optimum time for a vaccination day or week is during a trough in incidence between epidemic

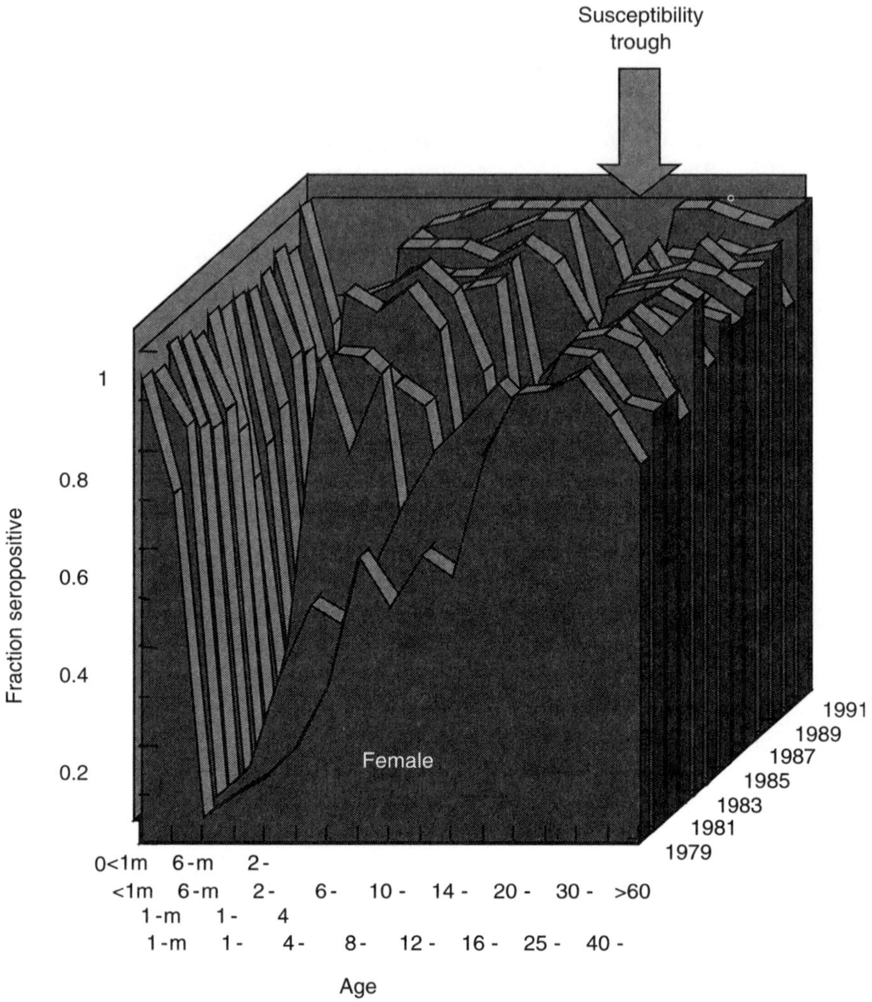

FIGURE 3-3 Herd immunity profile for rubella in Finland, recording the trough in susceptibility moving across the surface following the initiation of mass immunization in 1981. The *y*-axis records the fraction of a sample of sera collected from a population that are seropositive to the antigens of the rubella virus, stratified by host age and year of collection (Ukkonen, 1996).

cycles. Catch-up campaigns are especially valuable in developed countries, where they serve to mop up susceptible pockets within the population. However, it is important to recognize that any cessation or decline in effectiveness of either cohort or pulse programs will rapidly lead to a build-up of susceptibles, particularly in high birth rate communities. Increased susceptibility makes a population vulnerable to the reintroduction of infection from other countries or areas with lower vaccine coverage. Molecular epidemiological studies have revealed how travelers carry infections, such as measles and rubella, across continents, thereby creating short chains of transmission within susceptible pockets in highly vaccinated populations (Bellini and Rota, 1998).

Persistence or Eradication

Chains of transmission often persist even within highly vaccinated communities in developed countries. A number of factors create difficulties during the final push for the elimination of indigenous transmission. First, successful programs tend to increase the average age of infection. Consequently, cases of infection are often observed in clusters in older age classes (i.e., older than the age class for which immunization is first offered). Second, incidence increases in the younger age classes (i.e., younger than the age class for which immunization is first offered). Third, the synchrony of epidemics among different spatial locations decreases. Prior to widespread immunization, the epidemic cycles of most childhood viral and bacterial infections are highly correlated in different spatial settings within countries. However, synchrony decreases significantly as vaccine coverage rises, incidence falls, and inter-epidemic periods lengthen (Bolker and Grenfell, 1996). Controlling these minor epidemics may require that catch-up campaigns be timed differently.

Eradication is especially difficult when there is variation in vaccine uptake among regions, areas, or spatial locations. In developed countries, vaccine uptake in poor inner-city communities is often low. Pockets of low immunity, particularly if linked with overcrowding, poor public health care facilities, and high birth rates, provide reservoirs of infection for the sustenance of transmission. The ever-growing connectedness of urban centers across the world via air, road, and rail (even within Africa) suggests that continued immunization is necessary in all regions until vaccine uptake is uniformly high across the globe. Increased vaccine uptake reduces effective community size, which results in greater fade-out (i.e., a greater number of weeks during which there are no reported cases of infection) (see Figure 3-4).

Cost-Effectiveness of Mass Immunization

The main obstacles to eradication of measles and polio are often perceived to be financial. In today's world of rising health care costs, where many different interventions are possible in both developed and developing countries, cost-effectiveness is a major factor to consider when deciding which intervention to use. An increasing number of vaccines are available

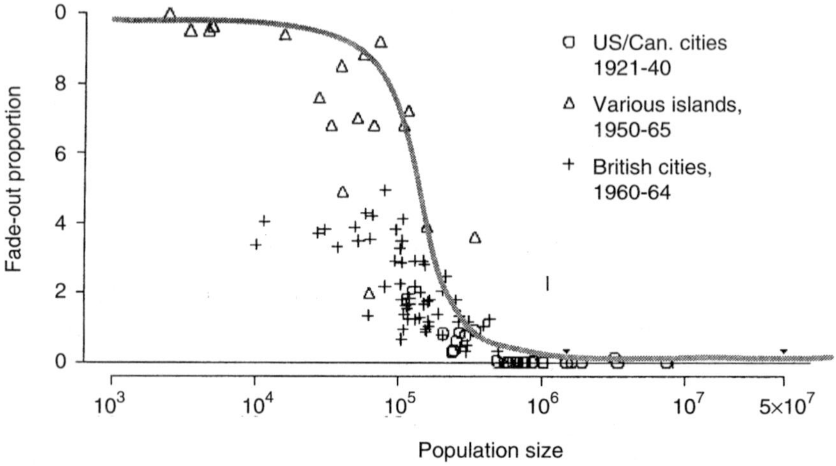

FIGURE 3-4 Critical community size for measles, defined as the population size at which fade-out (proportion of weeks in a year when no cases reported) of cases rises rapidly to approach unity.

for both viral (e.g., varicella) and bacterial infections (e.g., pneumococcal infections). Pharmaceutical companies and government health agencies often use cost-benefit analyses to determine which vaccine to use. However, these analyses tend to grossly underestimate the benefit of vaccination programs, because the current health economic methods of analysis typically only take into account the direct effects of immunization on the vaccinated individual. In practice, immunization has important indirect effects as well because it decreases transmission among those still unvaccinated. The magnitude of these indirect benefits increases rapidly as overall vaccine coverage increases and, as illustrated in Figure 3-5, may comprise a significant fraction of the overall benefit. The magnitude of the indirect benefit is calculated in a way that takes into account the impact of immunization on transmission success as a function of vaccination coverage. The time frame over which benefit is calculated (i.e., the number of years) is critical for an accurate assessment of cost versus benefit.

Morbidity Induced by Immunization

All vaccines carry a small risk of adverse effects in the immunized patient (Peltola and Heinonen, 1986). When the disease is common, risk of serious morbidity from infection is many orders of magnitude greater than risk associated with immunization. The values of the two risks converge when vaccine coverage approaches the level required to block local trans-

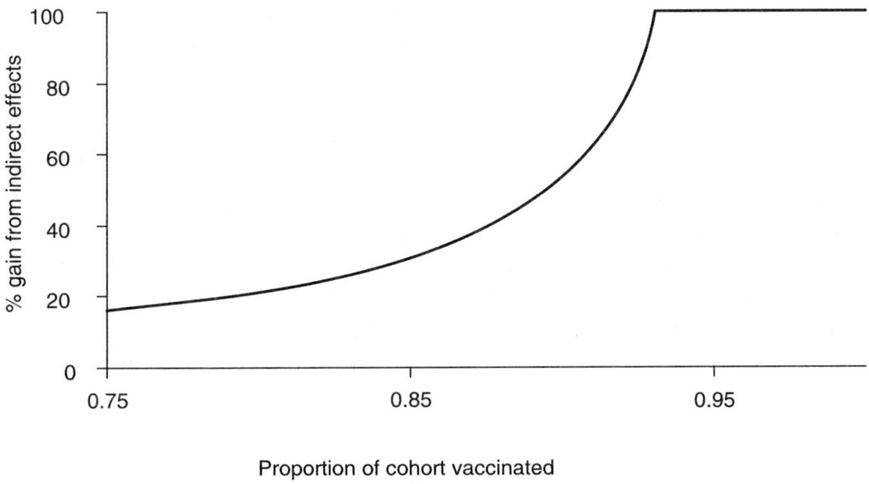

FIGURE 3-5 The indirect benefits arising from a mass measles vaccination program.

mission. When the disease is very rare or eliminated, the risk from vaccination is greater than the risk of morbidity from infection. At this point, the optimum strategy for each parent is to persuade every one else to immunize their children but not vaccinate their own!

One way around the inevitable conflict between individual and community interests is to pass legislation requiring vaccination before attending school or entering a country. For example, the United States requires evidence of immunization for school attendance (unless there are contraindications for individuals). Such legislation has found little favor in Europe, but recent events may change this. For example, in the United Kingdom, in the past few years unfounded reports of an association between MMR vaccination and autism in children has resulted in a significant decline in vaccine uptake in the last two years. The spurious correlation arises from the fact that the average age of onset of autism prior to wide-scale immunization was around two years of age, which is also the current average age at first immunization. Very recent detailed studies have shown no association between vaccination and autism (Kaye et al., 2001). The net effect of the decline in vaccine uptake in the UK will probably be upcoming measles epidemics on a scale not seen since the late 1960s.

Evolution

Mass vaccination at high levels of uptake imposes a very significant selective pressure on infectious agents by favoring rare antigenic variants whose major antigens, or major epitopes on defined antigens, are not adequately captured in the antigenic constituents of current vaccines. This problem has not arisen for measles, rubella, varicella, or mumps. However, antigenic variability in wild-type populations of hepatitis B, as well as several bacterial infections being targeted by new vaccines, is high. Greater antigenic variability allows for more opportunity for selection for rare variants. For infections that are targets for local elimination, surveillance based on molecular epidemiological approaches is essential for tracking evolutionary changes that might result in mutants prospering within highly vaccinated populations. Currently, surveillance is available only for infections, such as influenza, for which vaccine development depends on the identification of the dominant antigenic variants circulating in any given year.

Conclusion

Much has been written in recent years about the prospects for the worldwide eradication of infections such as measles and polio. Indeed, the title of this meeting hints at future success. However, it is far from clear that success is just around the corner. A particular problem with both measles and polio is the high transmissibility of both infections in densely populated urban areas. The average age of infection is low for both diseases, and in most urban communities vaccine coverage must be greater than 95% in order to block indigenous transmission. In contrast, smallpox had a high average age of infection prior to wide-scale vaccination, even in densely populated areas, and was much less transmissible than either polio or measles (Fenner et al., 1988).

In developed countries, mass vaccination will probably have to be maintained at very high levels for quite a while in order to protect against reintroductions from areas where poverty, human conflict, or absence of political will impedes high coverage. The only alternative to this would be demanding that travelers entering countries where the eradication of indigenous transmission has been achieved (or will be in the near future) show evidence of vaccination (e.g., saliva-based serology) as a condition for entry. The ever-increasing mobility of populations is a key factor in any elimination strategy. It must be assumed that if a directly transmitted infection persists in any corner of the globe, it will eventually find its way back into highly vaccinated populations if herd immunity is allowed to decline.

In highly vaccinated communities, the most immediate challenges to effective mass vaccination are public and professional complacency and the increasing publicity about adverse reactions to vaccination. For example, young physicians and health care workers in developed countries who have never witnessed measles infections may be unable to diagnose rare cases and may not be diligent in recommending immunization to all their patients. Similarly, in countries where infections are now rare, many young parents are unfamiliar with the serious morbidity associated with infection and may instead be influenced by the publicized risks associated with vaccination. Constant vigilance and effective education are essential.

ERROR, HUBRIS, AND MALICE

C.J. Peters, M.D.

Professor, Departments of Pathology and Microbiology and Immunology
University of Texas Medical Branch, Galveston, TX

The interruption of viral transmission associated with viral disease eradication requires a high vaccination coverage of the human population, a vaccine that eliminates transmission in a certain region for the duration of intensive immunization, and an effective assay for the virus and its antibodies. The biological basis of these requirements necessitates a thorough understanding of the viruses being targeted for eradication.

An Anthropocentric Classification of Viruses

Viruses can be divided into three groups: "true" human viruses that are maintained through chronic or latent infection; viruses that circulate in nature and infect humans from an extrahuman reservoir; and viruses transmitted among humans, without animal reservoir.

"True" human viruses that are maintained through chronic or latent infection (e.g., herpesvirus and polyomaviruses).

These viruses are believed to have shared a long co-evolutionary history with primates. They are generally not highly pathogenic except in immunosuppressed hosts. Their tight linkage to humans over the centuries makes their eradication virtually impossible, even though many of these viruses have been eliminated in certain non-human primate populations. For example, herpes-free colonies of rhesus macaques exist, and it is probably possible to generate lentivirus-free Old World monkey colonies.

Viruses that circulate in nature and infect humans from an extrahuman reservoir.

These viruses often have complicated transmission cycles which create more opportunities for interruption but also more strategies for survival. (Viruses, such as dengue, that have a non-human cycle but have adapted well to humans may be somewhat ambiguous.)

Even though several vector-borne parasitic diseases, such as malaria, are readily transmitted over long distances, most arthropod-borne virus introductions fail outside their usual range. There are some exceptions to this, such as the yellow fever and dengue viruses, and possibly the West Nile and Japanese encephalitis viruses. Also, even though Rift Valley fever failed to establish itself outside its sub-Saharan habitat after a large epidemic in Egypt in 1977, it continues to threaten distant spread. Successful long-distance introductions seem to involve vectors that are very adaptable and readily transportable (e.g., *Aedes aegypti* and *Culex pipiens*), or viruses (e.g., Venezuelan equine encephalitis and Rift Valley fever virus) that can be readily transmitted by multiple mosquito species in the presence of high viremias in imported vertebrate reservoirs (horses, sheep, and cattle).

One strategy for regional disease eradication involves eliminating human-virus contact, such as has been attempted for triatomid-Chagas or tsetse-trypanosomiasis parasite-vectors. These attempts have been relatively successful, but they fail when public health and social underpinnings collapse. Furthermore, other elements may intercede to change the dynamic; for example, the increased incidence of human AIDS has drastically altered the transmission of visceral leishmaniasis in the Americas.

Another strategy for eliminating viruses that are transmitted via arthropods involves eliminating the arthropod vector, since most arboviruses are highly dependent on a single arthropod species. For example, malaria transmission was reduced in Brazil by eliminating introduced *Anopheles gambiae* from South America, and urban yellow fever has been controlled by regional elimination of *Ae. aegypti*. However, *Ae. aegypti* ultimately recurred for multiple reasons, and there is still a risk of reintroduction of the highly efficient malaria vector, *An. gambiae*. This strategy requires a strong will and methodologies that are in short supply. Total elimination of a vector is unlikely.

Arthropod-borne viruses could be eradicated by eliminating their reservoirs. This is rarely desirable, however, except through vaccination of susceptibles, which is how Venezuelan equine encephalitis was eliminated from North, Central, and much of South America in the 1970s.

Rodent-borne viruses (e.g., lymphocytic choriomeningitis virus in *Mus musculus* or Seoul virus in *Rattus*) are notably resistant to control strategies because they are tightly linked to their host species and may move long distances as their hosts invade new geographic areas. The total elimination of a rodent species is generally neither desirable nor feasible. A possible elimination strategy involves selectively immunizing rodent populations that come into close contact with humans. For example, genetically engineered grains containing protective genes against hantaviruses could be used to make homes safe against deer mouse-borne hantaviruses. In situations such as lentivirus infection of humans, multiple introductions indicate that adaptation and spread of the virus among humans over time is probably more relevant than any unique primate-human contact. This suggests that even though limiting primate-human interactions is impractical and would never be completely successful, surveillance of subsequent human spread could be an efficient mechanism to limit lentivirus interspecies adaptation.

Viruses transmitted among humans, without animal reservoir.

With viruses transmitted among humans without an animal reservoir and that do not chronically infect their usual human host (e.g., measles, polio, and smallpox); intervention strategies involve using highly effective vaccines to break the mandatory human link in transmission. All viruses currently under consideration for eradication are of this type.

Post-Eradication Challenges

Major challenges for post-eradication strategies include:

1. *How can we assure that laboratory-preserved virus stocks and vaccine strains that could potentially revert to wild-type are eliminated or safely contained*? This includes vials clearly labeled "measles" or "polio," samples from respiratory disease patients who may have had measles, stool samples from patients who have had suspected enterovirus infections or asymptomatic poliovirus infection and so on. These samples are often retained through inertia but may also be archived for future study when new technology or information becomes available. Samples that may have initially yielded negative results are often sources for the identification of important "new" diseases or their agents (e.g., Fort Bragg fever and Pontiac fever). Destruction of samples can be difficult even under the most cooperative situation. Some viruses, such as poliovirus, can survive in mechanical freezers and liquid nitrogen repositories for a very long time.

2. *Are the viruses really "gone"*? We are entering an era in which small viral genomes can be synthesized and converted to infectious agents. Soon, even larger viruses will likely be synthesized from sequence information or clones. Thus, an apparently eradicated virus may be recovered in infectious form to threaten humanity anew.

3. *How will we continue research on important scientific questions that have already received enormous investment in terms of human effort and laboratory observation over the years*? For example, we scarcely understand the pathogenesis of the large, complicated smallpox virus, the exquis-

ite structure-function relationships of the much simpler poliovirus, and the subtle interactions of measles with the immune system. Unraveling these important infectious disease problems will require increased investment in containment laboratories, use of alternate virus-host systems for study, or investigations limited to a few expressed proteins. Control over virus gene distribution is problematic because many sequences have already been published, and the technology to reconstitute virtually any virus will soon be available.

4. *How will continued vaccine availability, testing, and a surge capacity be assured?* This may be only a short-term problem since eradication should eliminate the need for these. Repositories of vaccine could be retained to deal with short-term emergencies. Contemporary vaccine technology will still be available because uncertainties about eradication and ongoing research will provide a need. However, there will quickly come a time when there will no longer be a capacity to manufacture vaccine. The possible future needs, including surge capacity, should be provided for in long-term eradication plans, although the possible financial underpinnings of this requirement are unclear.

5. *Are there solutions to potential long-term problems with vaccines that could arise during post-eradication?* Recently, for example, the possibilities of the use of the smallpox virus in biowarfare or bioterrorism have necessitated the production of new vaccine stocks. But the technology is outdated. After the eradication of smallpox, vaccine stocks decayed, vaccine program infrastructure deteriorated, standards of vaccine production changed, and risk-benefit considerations shifted. It is too late to develop an improved vaccine because the immune basis for protection has never been defined, plus it is impossible to test a vaccine after eradication. Fortunately, simple cell culture adaptation of vaccinia virus is highly likely to produce a vaccine with qualities similar to the classical vaccine.

Another potential post-eradication need for vaccine or possibly anti-virals is the prevention or treatment of immunosuppressed individuals who develop vaccinia or vaccine-related poliovirus infection. In the case of poliovirus, for example, control would probably be impossible with the Salk vaccine because it is not known to reliably interrupt transmission and control with the Sabin vaccine would expose the borders of the vaccinated groups to partially reverted virus transmission. A subunit or vectored vaccine with mucosal efficacy would be invaluable; it would prevent the risk of reversion to virulence associated with attenuated vaccines, and it would eliminate the possibility of residual live virus being present in inactivated vaccines (a known problem for several viruses, including poliovirus and the animal foot and mouth disease virus). More data need to be gathered, ideally using non-human primate models if not humans, to show how effective human vaccines can be produced without propagating infectious virus.

Extinction

We live in a period of unprecedented extinction of plants, animals, and probably viruses. It is noteworthy that inventories of biodiversity rarely take viruses into account. Many feel it is not worth arguing over elimination of a virus that only spreads among humans and has severe adverse health effects. If an infectious virus does go extinct but information is still needed that requires a viral genome or even a live virus, viral genes could readily be synthesized from nucleic acid sequences. The virus itself could probably be recovered from sequences or clones.

For viruses maintained in nature with only incidental human infection, the consequences of extinction are unclear. Ecological systems are complex, interactive, and subtle, and loss of a key species can have important ramifications for many other species. The impact of most viruses on ecology, apart from human infection, has received little direct attention. For example, the fitness effect of hantaviruses or arenaviruses on their rodent reservoirs has not been assessed beyond simple trap-release data. However, a number of parasite studies indicate that these agents have considerable potential to regulate their host populations, which suggests caution in any attempt to eliminate a given virus. Total elimination of an animal vector or reservoir would be even more problematic.

Habitat destruction drives some important reservoirs to extinction, thereby facilitating control of disease. For example, the yellow fever situation in the Americas will be expected to improve with extensive deforestation and loss of its reservoir's habitat. The chimpanzee reservoir of the HIV-1 precursor virus will also likely be exterminated through the same mechanism.

Infectious agents themselves may participate in extinctions. For example, trypanosome parasites have eliminated cattle from parts of Africa, and the African horse sickness virus has eliminated unvaccinated equines from certain areas. Small populations with limited genetic variability (e.g., cheetahs and viral peritonitis) or in close contact with diseased populations (e.g., lions infected with distemper or tuberculosis) may be at an increased risk for extinction from viruses. Still, there is no known example of a virus having eliminated its host species when the host species is otherwise healthy in terms of ecology and habitat.

Laboratory Containment

Containment has two basic elements: protection of the environment from microbes in the laboratory, and protection of the workers (or bystanders) from infection or contamination. The former is essential to containing infectious agents when the external environment is receptive to infection, and the latter is important when the worker serves as a route of escape for the agent.

The use of established standards, such as BSL-4 or BSL-3, as a form of protection of both the environment and the laboratory worker has generally been very successful. These standards have been applied to many hazardous viruses in the past and have not resulted in any environmental problems and only infrequent worker infections.

It is generally recognized that BSL-4 is more stringent than BSL-3, but the differences are not well appreciated. BSL-3 is used for highly aerosol-infectious agents that cause human disease. For example, lymphocytic choriomeningitis virus is classified as BSL-3 because of its capability to efficiently infect the laboratory worker with low concentrations of small particle aerosols. BSL-4 agents are also aerosol infections but they cause severe human disease for which there is no established vaccine or therapy. Lassavirus is an example of a BSL-4 agent. Other viruses that cause similarly severe diseases but are not infectious by aerosols (except by massive exposures) can be used at BSL-2. In BSL-2 aerosol exposure is minimized by using special precautions (for example, a laminar flow biosafety cabinet) while handling concentrated virus or performing operations such as centrifugation that can generate high concentrations of aerosols. In BSL-3 all manipulations of virus are performed inside a biosafety cabinet or using other methods to contain aerosols.

There are several differences between BSL-4 and BSL-3 containment. Most obviously, BSL-4 workers are encased in a flexible plastic "space suit" with their own air supply, or the viruses are segregated in a sealed negative pressure glove box. The suit serves to protect the worker from infection and in addition can be surface decontaminated when the worker leaves the BSL-4 environment. BSL-4 mechanical systems are more redundant, particularly those used for air flow (e.g., two fans are used with a back-up generator, and the air passes through two HEPA filters). Also, BSL-4 sewage discharge is sterilized.

Intermediate systems that incorporate more controls than BSL-3 but are not as stringent as BSL-4 are usually referred to as "BSL-3+." This terminology is ambiguous and dangerous. The facilities are usually not carefully evaluated for the exact safeguards that are needed and, in the absence of a defined standard, are not carefully controlled. Additionally, the staff is often inexperienced; it must be emphasized that even with BSL-4, proper attitude, safety training, and experience are the most important elements of containment.

Viruses like polio and smallpox have sustained continuous interhuman transmission for centuries. Their eradication may present a situation unlike any of our previous experience with biological containment. In the case of smallpox, however, the use of laboratories with filtered air and shower-out, coupled with careful vaccination of the workers, has successfully contained the virus during times in which population immunity has been low. But to contain smallpox at the BSL-4 level reflects an "Ebola-doomsday-Frankenstein" mentality and the current trend to over-contain. With regards to containment of the poliovirus, factors to consider will include glove precautions, the comparatively high stability of the virus, and the consequences of any manipulations that might be done with the virus.

Genetic Modification

The age of bioengineering started with a very conservative approach which relied on experimental evidence from *Escherichia coli*, a well-understood, innocuous organism, and careful oversight from the Recombinant Advisory Committee. Certain experiments with toxins or expression of physiological active molecules have been avoided. This experience has given us a tremendous amount of confidence with several engineered systems and has enormously loosened oversight. For example, careful work with the La Crosse virus and its relatives showed that reassortant viruses are no more virulent than their most virulent partner.

This idea about the virulence of recombinant viruses seems to be a reasonable principle at this time; however, recent data raise some important questions. Reverse genetics has allowed the laboratory construction of a number of different viruses. Common sense suggests that certain experiments (e.g., such as reconstruction of the 1918 influenza virus) would be unreasonable. But would the poliovirus, for example, be a target for the virus equivalent of a "hacker"? Reverse genetics has also allowed the construction of chimeric viruses with surprisingly high fitnesses. Orthopoxviruses have proven to be useful and safe vectors for many genes, but the recent report of enhanced murine virulence of ectromelia expressing an IL4 gene is disquieting. Should there be more oversight of or discussion about these experiments?

Biological Warfare or Terrorism

This increasingly disquieting aspect of modern life must not be ignored. Reconstitution of poliovirus, release of hidden stocks of smallpox virus, and other mischief are all possible. Although they would limit the damage, precautions may not completely protect us (particularly against blackmail). We should actively pursue intelligence and law enforcement programs aimed at preventing bioterrorism with these agents. However, these programs should be designed in such a way that active research on the viruses can continue.

Conclusion

Some research objectives in the post-eradication, and particularly in the post-vaccination period, may need to be abandoned. If they are unique to the agent in question, they may not be sufficiently important to justify continuation in a highly contained laboratory for an indefinite period. More general research may require investing in other virus-host systems that do not require expensive containment and do not carry the small but inescapable risk of virus escape. By allowing expression of only a limited number of viral genes, investigations of specific phenomena could continue without the use of infectious viruses.

Containment of the eradicated organisms should be based on staff training and attitude, engineering redundancy, shower-out facilities, control of effluent air and waste, and previous experience with the agent. Whenever possible, evidence should be collected from realistic settings in order to determine containment needs. Knee-jerk assertions that BSL-4 containment is necessary or sufficient should be avoided.

Post-eradication strategies should involve consideration of how to deal with recrudescence of disease for at least several decades. This will require stockpiling a modest amount of a proven vaccine, renewing the stockpiles over time, and providing the capacity for surge production. The possibility of reversion of live-attenuated vaccines, as well as the possibility of residual live virus in inactivated vaccines, should also be considered. Ideally, the vaccine will be derived from genes from the eradicated virus but will not involve the use of inactivated or attenuated immunogens from the virus. This type of vaccine would make containment during production easier.

NATURAL SIV RESERVOIRS AND HUMAN ZOONOTIC RISK: CHALLENGES TO DISEASE ERADICATION

Beatrice H. Hahn, M.D.

Professor, Department of Medicine and Microbiology
University of Alabama at Birmingham, Birmingham, AL

Evidence of simian immunodeficiency virus (SIV) infection has been reported for 26 different species of African non-human primates. Two of these viruses, SIVcpz from chimpanzees and SIVsm from sooty mangabeys, have crossed the species barrier to humans on multiple occasions, generating human immunodeficiency virus types 1 and 2 (HIV-1 and HIV-2), respectively. Thus, an important public health concern is whether and to what extent humans continue to be exposed to SIV, and whether such exposure has led to additional zoonotic transmissions. Such transmissions could undermine AIDS vaccine efforts and other strategies aimed at HIV eradication.

Emerging infectious diseases represent a major threat to public health. The disease with the greatest global impact to have emerged recently is the acquired immunodeficiency syndrome (AIDS). First recognized in the early 1980s, AIDS represents the end-stage of infection with either human immunodeficiency lentivirus type 1 (HIV-1) or 2 (HIV-2). While HIV-2 is virtually restricted to west Africa (van der Loeff and Aaby, 1999), HIV-1 has spread globally and is estimated to have caused over 50 million infections worldwide (UNAIDS, 2000). Although antiretroviral therapies have slowed disease progression and reduced mortality, these treatments do not eradicate infection and are inaccessible in most developing countries. With 5 million new infections estimated annually worldwide, HIV/AIDS is now the leading cause of death in sub-Saharan Africa (UNAIDS, 2000). A vaccine to prevent HIV infection and/or disease will ultimately be needed to control the explosive spread of HIV/AIDS, especially in the developing world.

The two types of human AIDS viruses, HIV-1 and HIV-2, are both of zoonotic origin (Hahn et al., 2000). Analysis of available sequence data indicates that HIV-1 is comprised of three distinct virus groups (termed M, N, and O), with the predominant M group consisting of nine sequence subtypes (A–D, F–H, J, K) (Kuiken et al., 1999). Similarly, HIV-2 strains have been found to be comprised of seven distinct phylogenetic lineages, designated subtypes A–G (Kuiken et al., 1999). Current phylogenetic evidence indicates that the SIV counterparts of HIV were introduced into the human population on multiple occasions (Hahn et al., 2000; Sharp et al., 2001). Yet, HIV-1 group M viruses, which are responsible for the great majority of all HIV infections worldwide, appear to have arisen from just one cross-species transmission event (Sharp et al., 2001). This highlights the potential significance of even a single primate lentiviral transmission from primates to humans and illustrates the importance of surveillance of human and primate populations for novel SIV infections.

African primates represent an extremely large reservoir of lentiviruses with the potential for infecting other species, including humans. A total of 26 different primate species are now known to harbor SIV (Hahn et al., 2000; Peeters et al., 2001). The primate lentiviruses for which full-length genomic sequences are available fall into six major, approximately equidistant phylogenetic lineages (Courgnaud et al., 2001; Hahn et al., 2000):

1. SIVcpz from chimpanzees (Pan troglodytes), together with HIV-1;
2. SIVsm from sooty mangabeys (Cercocebus atys), together with HIV-2 and SIVmac from macaques (several Macaca sp.);
3. SIVagm from four species of African green monkeys (Chlorocebus sp.);

4. SIVsyk from Sykes' monkeys (Cercopithecus albogularis);
5. SIVlhoest from l'Hoest monkeys (Cercopithecus lhoesti), SIVsun from sun-tailed monkeys (Cercopithecus solatus), and SIVmnd1 from a mandrill (Mandrillus sphinx); and
6. SIVcol from colobus monkeys (Colobus guereza).

Partial sequences are available for a number of additional SIVs, but their phylogenetic relationships remain to be fully resolved.

Phylogenetic analyses have shown that all viruses from any one simian species are generally much more closely related to each other than to viruses from other species (Hahn et al., 2000). SIV transfers between different primate species in the wild have been documented; however, the frequency of such transmission events, the clinical outcomes, and the factors required for establishing new primate lentiviral infections are unknown. For example, transmissions of SIVagm to sympatric patas monkeys and baboons have been reported in the wild (Bibollet-Ruche et al., 1996; Jin et al., 1994a; van Rensburg et al., 1998). Additionally, the analysis of several complex recombinant SIV strains, including SIVrcm infecting red-capped mangabeys (*Cercocebus torquatus*) (Georges-Courbot et al., 1998), SIVmnd2 infecting mandrills (*Mandrillus sphinx*) (Souquiere et al., 2001), and SIVagmSab infecting sabaeus monkeys (*Chlorocebus sabaeus*) (Jin et al., 1994b) have provided indirect evidence of cross-species transmission (Hahn et al., 2000).

Strains of SIV closely related to HIV-2 have been isolated from sooty mangabeys (*Cercocebus atys*) and three different macaque (*Macaca* sp.) species. Only a few macaques, all in captivity in North America, have been found to carry these viruses; these species are not naturally infected with SIV in the Asian wild. In contrast, SIVsm has been isolated from wild sooty mangabeys in West Africa (Chen et al., 1996). HIV-2 is only endemic in West Africa, and it seems clear that SIVsm has been transmitted to humans there, as well as to macaques in captivity. Detailed consideration of the phylogenetic relationships among SIVsm and HIV-2 strains indicates that cross-species transmission to humans has occurred on at least five different occasions (Chen et al., 1997; Gao et al., 1992; Gao et al., 1994). However, recent analyses of new SIVsm strains strongly suggest that each of the seven HIV-2 subtypes likely arose from separate cross-species transmission events (Sharp et al., 2001).

Strains of SIV closely related to HIV-1 have only been isolated from chimpanzees (*Pan troglodytes*). Seven SIVcpz-infected chimpanzees have thus far been identified, all of which were captured as young orphans (Corbet et al., 2000; Gao et al., 1999; Peeters et al., 1989; Peeters et al., 1992). Of these seven, one clearly acquired his infection in captivity from a naturally infected cage mate (Corbet et al., 2000). The other six are either known or believed to represent natural infections, and five of them have been identified in chimpanzees from west central Africa (*P. t. troglodytes*). A sixth strain was isolated from a wild-caught chimpanzee of unknown geographic origin which was classified as a *P. t. schweinfurthii* on the basis of mtDNA analyses (Gao et al., 1999; Peeters et al., 1992). All three groups of HIV-1 are significantly more closely related to the five SIVcpz(P.t.t.) isolates than to the one SIVcpz(P.t.s.) strain, indicating that the cross-species transmissions that gave rise to all three groups of HIV-1 (M, N, and O) occurred in west central Africa (Gao et al., 1999). HIV-1 groups N and O viruses are essentially restricted to west central Africa (Mauclere et al., 1997; Simon et al., 1998), and chimpanzee and group N human viruses from Cameroon form a unique subcluster in phylogenetic trees, implicating this country as the likely site of origin for HIV-1 group N (Corbet et al., 2000; Simon et al., 1998). Although HIV-1 group M is spreading globally, the greatest diversity of group M viruses has been found in the western parts of the Democratic Republic of Congo (i.e., Kinshasa), which is consistent with this being the region of the initial group M expansion (Vidal et al., 2000). Kinshasa is outside the range of chimpanzees, but it is close to the natural range of *P. t. troglodytes* and is by far the largest city in the region. Together, these findings provide compelling evidence that HIV-1 arose as a consequence of three independent SIVcpz transmissions from naturally infected chimpanzees in west central Africa.

Although the routes and circumstances of cross-species transmissions are unknown, it is believed that human infection with SIVcpz and SIVsm resulted from exposure to infected blood during the hunting and field dressing of animals, the preparation of primate meat for consumption, and bites and scratches from infected pets or wounded animals (Hahn et al., 2000). Given that humans throughout sub-Saharan Africa are in frequent contact with primate species other than chimpanzees and sooty mangabeys, the possibility of additional zoonotic transfers of primate lentiviruses must be considered. Indeed, a recent survey of bushmeat markets in Cameroon revealed that up to one-third of all primates offered for sale were SIV-infected (Peeters et al., 2001). Peeters and colleagues found that over 130 of 400 wild-caught monkeys from 13 different species had serum antibodies that cross-reacted with HIV-1 and/or HIV-2 antigens. PCR amplification of viral sequences confirmed SIV infection in a subset of these animals and revealed the existence of four new SIV lineages not previously known to infect primates in the wild. This study thus provided conclusive evidence that humans are routinely exposed to a wide variety of primate lentiviruses through the hunting and handling of SIV-infected primates.

Commercial logging represents an important economic activity in many west central African countries; it has led to road construction into remote forest areas, human migration, and the development of social and economic networks which support this industry (Auzel and Hardin, 2000; Geist, 1988; Wilkie et al., 2000). Hunters are now penetrating previously inaccessible forest areas and using modern weapons and a newly developed infrastructure to capture and transport bushmeat, including many primates, from remote areas to major city markets. These socioeconomic changes, combined with current data on SIV prevalence and genetic complexity in wild living primates, strongly suggest that the magnitude of human exposure to SIV has increased dramatically, as have the social and environmental conditions that support the emergence of new zoonotic infections.

It remains unknown whether SIVs other than SIVcpz and SIVsm have the ability to infect humans. Molecular evidence for such cross-species transmissions does not exist; however, such infections might have gone unrecognized. An example is the recent identification of a Cameroonian man who had an indeterminant HIV serology but reacted strongly with an SIVmnd V3 loop peptide (Souquiere et al., 2001). Although SIV infection was not confirmed in this individual, the finding suggests that at least some naturally occurring SIVs (other than SIVcpz and SIVsm) have the potential to infect humans. In fact, several recently reported SIV isolates (Georges-Courbet et al., 1998; Souquiere et al., 2001) replicate well in primary human lymphocytes *in vitro*, as do SIVcpz (Gao et al., 1999; Peeters et al., 1992) and SIVsm (Peeters et al., 1994). Thus, to determine whether additional zoonotic transmissions of SIVs have already occurred, screening assays that can reliably recognize and distinguish the wide variety of SIVs now known to infect wild-living primates will have to be developed.

It is also important to distinguish between the initial transmission of a new SIV and the many additional factors that promote secondary transmissions and, ultimately, epidemic spread in the human population. The factors that trigger epidemic outbreaks of newly introduced SIVs are unknown but could possibly involve situations where the recipient of a cross-species transmission event is already infected by an existing HIV. In these cases, superinfection and recombination could generate mosaic viruses of considerable genetic and biological complexity. Evidence that such events have taken place in primates has come from studies of SIVs infecting sabaeus monkeys (SIVagmSab), red-capped mangabeys (SIVrcm), and mandrills (SIVmnd2) (Georges-Courbet et al., 1998; Jin et al., 1994b; Souquiere et al., 2001). In each case, mosaic viruses comprised of different SIV lineages are widely distributed in their respective host species and thus represent cases where cross-species transmission and recombination have led to successful virus adaptation and dissemination, perhaps even outcompeting the previous incumbent SIVs. As the prevalence rates of HIV-1 group M viruses are rising in west central Africa, recombination of newly introduced SIVs with circulating HIVs has become a more probable scenario.

TABLE 3-1 SIV Reservoirs and Human Zoonotic Risk: Future Studies

Determine the full spectrum of SIV-infected non-human primates in equatorial Africa:

- Identify all SIV-infected primate species.
- Assess the prevalence, geographic distribution, and natural history of SIV infection in wild primate populations.
- Determine the frequencies, routes, and circumstances of primate-to-primate cross-species transmissions.

Characterize all major SIV lineages at the biological and molecular level:

- Determine the spectrum of SIV genetic and biological diversity.
- Molecularly clone and sequence representatives of all major SIV lineages.
- Characterize the origins and evolutionary history of the entire group of primate lentiviruses.

Determine to what extent humans are exposed to SIV and whether such exposure has led to additional zoonotic transmissions:

- Develop novel screening and confirmatory assays that can detect and distinguish the wide variety of SIV infections now known to exist in wild primate populations.
- Establish effective surveillance mechanisms for humans at risk for zoonotic infections.
- Elucidate the viral, host, and environmental factors that facilitate zoonotic transmission and promote subsequent epidemic spread.
- Monitor the emergence of HIV/SIV recombinants.

In summary, the current HIV-1 group M pandemic provides compelling evidence for the rapidity, stealth, and, ultimately, the extraordinary clinical impact that can result from even a single zoonotic transmission event. It is now clear that humans are routinely exposed to a plethora of primate lentiviruses through the hunting of primates, and that the magnitude and breadth of this exposure has previously been underestimated.

In light of these data, a complete and accurate assessment of all SIV-infected non-human primate species in geographic areas where these are abundant seems necessary (Table 3-1). Since most SIV-infected primates, especially the great apes, are endangered, strategies that avoid a further increase in hunting will need to be employed. Such strategies would rely on non-invasive methods, such as the use of urine and fecal samples to detect SIV-specific antibodies and viral nucleic acids (Santiago et al., 2001). Studies are also needed to determine whether transmission of simian lentiviruses other than SIVcpz and SIVsm to humans have already occurred. This will require the screening of human sera with diagnostic tests which can detect and distinguish a wide range of primate lentiviral infections.

Finally, the potential of recombination between currently circulating HIVs and newly introduced SIVs must be considered, and surveillance mechanisms must be established to detect their possible emergence. Such recombinants could evade susceptibility to vaccines that are based on only one virus group or subtype. Because experimental HIV vaccines will eventually be tested in countries worldwide, the occurrence of new zoonotic SIV infections and their possible impact on immunization efforts will need to be examined. The existence of a primate reservoir must be taken into account while planning future eradication strategies for HIV/AIDS.

VACCINE-ASSOCIATED CASES DUE TO IMMUNIZATION WITH LIVE VIRUS VACCINES

Jeffrey I. Cohen, M.D.

Head, Medical Virology Section, Laboratory of Clinical Investigation
National Institutes of Health, Bethesda, MD

Live virus vaccines, including those for smallpox, measles, and poliovirus, have dramatically reduced or in some cases eliminated disease caused by these viruses. As disease due to wild-type virus is eliminated, however, vaccine-associated cases become of increasing concern.

Vaccinia, which has been used for 200 years to prevent smallpox, can cause postvaccinal encephalitis, progressive vaccinia, eczema vaccinatum, and generalized vaccinia. In a national survey in 1968, about 300 of 14 million vaccinees suffered severe side effects, and 9 fatalities were reported. All but one of the fatalities were due to postvaccinal encephalitis or progressive vaccinia. Fatal cases of eczema vaccinatum have been reported in contacts of vaccinees. A case of severe generalized vaccinia occurred in a vaccinated asymptomatic HIV military recruit. The smallpox viral genome contains 150 genes that are very similar to vaccinia and 37 genes that are smallpox-specific or divergent from those in vaccinia. These latter genes frequently encode host-interactive proteins.

The vaccine strain of measles virus rarely causes disease. Vaccine virus has been detected in lung, liver, bone marrow, or brain tissues of only three patients who had severe disease after vaccination. One patient had HIV, one had severe combined immunodeficiency, and one had no known immunodeficiency. The latter two patients died from measles vaccination. The measles vaccine and wild-type virus share more than 95.5% of the same nucleotide sequences. The changes that are responsible for attenuation of the measles virus are unknown.

Vaccine-Associated Paralytic Poliomyelitis

The first reports of vaccine-associated paralytic poliomyelitis (VAPP) occurred shortly after the introduction of the oral polio vaccine (OPV). Since 1973, the number of VAPP cases has exceeded the number of cases of wild-type polio in the United States. From 1980–1989, VAPP was associated with 1 out of every 2.5 million doses of OPV in the United States. VAPP occurs primarily in unvaccinated or inadequately vaccinated persons, and more commonly in infants. In the United States from 1980 to 1995, about 40% of VAPP cases occurred in OPV recipients, 30% in close contacts, 25% in immunodeficient persons, and 5% were community acquired. The latter persons had not been recently vaccinated and were not known to be in direct contact with vaccine recipients. The percentage of patients in each risk group has remained fairly stable over time.

Immunodeficient patients have a 3,000- to 6,000-fold greater risk of developing VAPP. In one study (Sutter and Prevots, 1994), 96% of VAPP cases were due to B cell deficiency; the other 4% were due to long-term corticosteroid use. So far, there have been only two cases of VAPP associated with HIV. In Romania, but not in the United States, VAPP has been associated with increasing numbers of intramuscular injections given nine to thirty days before OPV.

Nucleotide sequencing indicates that less than 1% of OPV bases (polio is an RNA virus and does not have base pairs) differ from those of its neurovirulent parent. Only two or three base changes are needed for OPV type 2 (OPV2) or OPV3 to revert to neurovirulence, while several base changes are needed for OPV1. This coincides with the fact that OPV2 and OPV3 are isolated more frequently than OPV1 from patients with VAPP.

VAPP may be due to neurovirulent revertant viruses that develop during replication in the gastrointestinal tract, recombination between different strains of OPV, or recombination between OPV and wild-type strains. In one study, within 2 days of receiving OPV3, one of the attenuating mutations in the virus reverted to the wild-type sequence, and the shed virus was more neurovirulent (Evans et al., 1985).

When OPV was the preferred vaccine, there were eight to nine VAPP cases per year in the United States. After the initiation of a sequential regimen of inactivated poliovirus vaccine (IPV)-OPV, the number of cases declined to two to five per year. With an all IPV regimen, VAPP should be virtually eliminated. However, there is concern about the continued release of neurovirulent revertants of live OPV into the environment even after vaccination is terminated. Thus, VAPP may continue to occur for some finite period of time. Recently, two antibody-deficient patients with VAPP shed virus in their stool for over five years after their last vaccination. Comparison of the sequence of these viruses with that of OPV suggests that the viruses had been replicating in the patients for about ten years. However, most antibody-deficient patients probably shed virus for less than six months. In contrast, immunocompetent persons usually shed virus for less than three months.

Several studies have suggested that OPV has a limited circulation in the environment. In Cuba, for example, where OPV is administered for two months of the year, the virus has been detected for only 2 or 3 months after vaccinations (Ochoa and Lago, 1987). Similarly, VAPP cases in Romania have been closely associated with specific vaccination campaigns (Strebel et al., 1994). In most cases, sequencing of VAPP isolates shows greater than 99% similarity to OPV, indicating that the VAPP isolates have circulated for a very short period of time.

However, other studies show that neurovirulent forms of OPV can circulate at length. For example, analysis of the nucleotide sequence of OPV2 isolated from sewage in Israel suggested that the virus had been circulating for six years (Shulman et al., 2000). A similar study from Japan found neurovirulent virus in sewage and river water three months after OPV vaccination (Yoshida et al., 2000). These neurovirulent strains of OPV were not associated with VAPP in either of these two studies.

In Poland, from March to December 1968, there was an outbreak of poliovirus type 3 four months after vaccination with a live attenuated OPV3, USOL virus. There were 464 cases of paralytic disease. Nucleotide sequencing of isolates from seven epidemic cases, four healthy vaccinees, and one healthy contact all showed USOL-like viruses. The seven isolates exhibited a change in sequence associated with neurovirulence; none of the healthy vaccinees or contacts exhibited such a change.

A large number of cases of polio occurred in China from 1991 to 1993. Sequencing of isolates from 34 patients indicated that the virus was a recombinant derivative of wild-type polio type 1 and OPV1. Analysis of the sequenced viruses suggested that all of the recombinants were derived from a mixed infection of a single person with wild-type and OPV type 1. The recombinant virus spread rapidly over 2,200 kilometers in 3 years.

Recent outbreaks of paralytic polio have occurred due to circulating vaccine-derived poliovirus (cVDPV) in several areas, suggesting that neurovirulent revertants of OPV can persist. For example, from July to November 2000, 20 cases of cVDPV due to OPV1 occurred in the Dominican Republic and Haiti. About 85% of the patients were under six years of age, and all of the patients were either unvaccinated or inadequately vaccinated. The viral nucleotide sequence showed a 97% genetic similarity to OPV, suggesting that the virus had either circulated for two years in the area or had undergone prolonged replication in an immunodeficient person. The epidemic was rapidly terminated after intensive vaccination with OPV. A similar epidemic of cVDPV due to OPV2 occurred in 32 persons in

Egypt from 1988–1993. Analysis of the viral sequence suggested that the virus had circulated for 11 years. Like the Caribbean epidemic, vaccination coverage was low in Egypt during this time, and circulation of OPV-derived virus stopped when vaccine coverage increased. From March to July 2001, 3 cases of cVDPV occurred in the Philippines. These cases were due to virus derived from OPV1.

Conclusion

These VAPP cases emphasize (a) the need for continuing polio vaccination in polio-free areas until global eradication is achieved, (b) the necessity of continued surveillance for poliovirus and flaccid paralysis, (c) the need for additional information about duration of shedding and persistence of virus in the environment, and (d) the importance of global eradication of poliovirus.

Remaining questions, and possible answers, include the following:

1. *Will immunocompromised carriers of OPV continue to shed the virus into the environment?* Yes, but only for a limited time—most often weeks to months, but in some cases for up to as long as 10 years.
2. *What proportion of immunocompromised persons (including those with HIV) shed OPV for prolonged periods of time?* Probably less than 10% of antibody-deficient patients shed virus for long periods of time; the percentage is probably lower among HIV-infected patients since they often retain the ability to produce antibodies.
3. *How long will neurovirulent revertants of OPV be shed into the environment?* Based on results from sewage studies in Japan and Israel, OPV can be detected for up to nearly five years after vaccination.
4. *What is the threshold rate of vaccine coverage needed to suppress circulation of OPV, and upon what does the rate depend?* The rate is probably similar to that required to prevent circulation of wild-type polio, and it probably depends on the strain of OPV, population density, level of hygiene, and climate.
5. *How long can OPV circulate in populations, and how transmissible is it?* OPV can circulate for 11 years according to the Egyptian outbreak of polio associated with OPV, and 2 years according to the Caribbean outbreak.
6. *Should IPV be given for a period of time after OPV is discontinued to allow clearing of virus from shedders?* Yes, if possible, especially since infants have the highest risk for VAPP and will not be immune when vaccination is stopped.
7. *How long should intensive surveillance be continued after IPV is*

stopped? Probably at least 10 years, in view of the long shedding period and the recent occurrence of polio due to circulating vaccine-related virus.

8. *What is the best way to detect circulating OPV and respond to outbreaks?* Intensive surveillance for cases of acute flaccid paralysis and poliovirus is required, and further research is needed.

REFERENCES

Agur Z, Cojocaru L, Mazor G, Anderson RM, and Danon YL. 1993. Pulse mass measles vaccination across age cohorts. *Proceedings of the National Academy of Sciences* 90:11698–11702.

Anderson RM. 1994. Populations, infectious disease and immunity: A very nonlinear world. *Philosophical Transactions of the Royal Society of London, Series B* 346:457–505.

Anderson RM and May RM. 1990. Immunization and herd immunity. *Lancet* 335:641–645.

Anderson RM and May RM. 1992. *Infectious Diseases of Humans: Dynamics and Control.* Oxford: University of Oxford Press.

Anderson RM, Donnelly CA, and Gupta S. 1997. Vaccine design, evaluation, and community-based use for antigenically variable infectious agents. *Lancet* 350:1466–1470.

Auzel P and Hardin R. 2000. Colonial history, concessionary politics, and collaborative management of Equatorial African rain forests. Pp. 21–38 in Hunting and Bushmeat Utilization in the African Rain Forest, M Bakarr, G Da Fonseca, W Konstant, R Mittermeier, and K Painemilla, eds. Washington, D.C.: Advances in Applied Biodiversity Science Series, Conservation International.

Bellini WJ and Rota PA. 1998. Genetic diversity of wild-type measles viruses: Implications for global measles elimination programs. *Emerging Infectious Diseases* 4:29–35.

Bibollet-Ruche F, Galat-Luong A, Cuny G, Sarni-Manchado P, Galat G, Durand JP, Pourrut X, and Veas F. 1996. Simian immunodeficiency virus infection in a patas monkey (*Erythrocebus patas*): Evidence for cross-species transmission from African green monkeys (*Cercopithecus aethiops sabaeus*) in the wild. *The Journal of General Virology* 77:773–781.

Bolker BM and Grenfell BT. 1996. Impact of vaccination on the spatial correlation and persistence of measles dynamics. *Proceedings of the National Academy of Sciences* 93:12648–12653.

Bottiger M, Christenson B, Romanus V, Taranger J, and Strandell A. 1987. Swedish experience of two-dose vaccination program aiming at eliminating measles, mumps, and rubella. *British Medical Journal* 295:1264–1267.

Chen Z, Telfer P, Gettie A, Reed P, Zhang L, Ho DD, and Marx PA. 1996. Genetic characterization of new West African simian immunodeficiency virus SIVsm: geographic clustering of household-derived SIV strains with human immunodeficiency virus type 2 subtypes and genetically diverse viruses from a single feral sooty mangabey troop. *Journal of Virology* 70:3617–3627.

Chen Z, Luckay A, Sodora DL, Telfer P, Reed P, Gettie A, Kanu JM, Sadek RF, Yee J, Ho DD, Zhang L, and Marx PA. 1997. Human immunodeficiency virus type 2 (HIV-2) seroprevalence and characterization of a distinct HIV-2 genetic subtype from the natural range of simian immunodeficiency virus-infected sooty mangabeys. *Journal of Virology* 71:3953–3960.

Corbet S, Muller-Trutwin MC, Versmisse P, Delarue S, Ayouba A, Lewis J, Brunak S, Martin P, Brun-Vezinet F, Simon F, Barre-Sinoussi F, and Mauclere P. 2000. Env sequences of simian immunodeficiency viruses from chimpanzees in Cameroon are strongly related to those of human immunodeficiency virus group N from the same geographic area. *Journal of Virology* 74:529–534.

Courgnaud V, Pourrut X, Bibollet-Ruche F, Mpoudi-Ngole E, Bourgeois A, Delaporte E, and Peeters M. 2001. Characterization of a novel simian immunodeficiency virus from Guereza Colobus (*Colobus guereza*) in Cameroon: A new lineage in the nonhuman primate lentivirus family. *Journal of Virology* 75:857–866.

de Quadros CA, Olive JM, Hersh BS, Strassburg MA, Henderson DA, Brandling-Bennett D, and Alleyne GA. 1996. Measles elimination in the Americas: Evolving strategies. *Journal of the American Medical Association* 275:224–229.

Evans DM, Dunn G, Minor PD, Schild GC, Cann AJ, Stanway G, Almond JW, Currey K, and Maizel JV Jr. 1985. Increased neurovirulence associated with a single nucleotide change in a noncoding region of the Sabin type 3 poliovaccine genome. *Nature* 314(6011):548–550.

Fenner F, Henderson DA, Arita I, Jezek Z, and Ladnyi ID. 1988. *Smallpox and Its Eradication*. Geneva: World Health Organization.

Gao F, Yue L, White AT, Pappas PG, Barchue J, Hanson AP, Greene BM, Sharp PM, Shaw GM, and Hahn BH. 1992. Human infection by genetically diverse SIVsm-related HIV-2 in west Africa. *Nature* 358:495–499.

Gao F, Yue L, Robertson DL, Hill SC, Hui H, Biggar RJ, Neequaye AE, Whelan TM, Ho DD, Shaw GM, Sharp PM, and Hahn BH. 1994. Genetic diversity of human immunodeficiency virus type 2: Evidence for distinct sequence subtypes with differences in virus biology. *Journal of Virology* 68:7433–7447.

Gao F, Bailes E, Robertson DL, Chen Y, Rodenburg CM, Michael SF, Cummins LB, Arthur LO, Peeters M, Shaw GM, Sharp PM, and Hahn BH. 1999. Origin of HIV-1 in the chimpanzee *Pan troglodytes troglodytes*. *Nature* 397:436–441.

Geist V. 1988. How markets for wildlife meat and parts, and the sale of hunting privileges, jeopardize wildlife conservation. *Conservation Biology* 2:15–26.

Georges-Courbot MC, Lu CY, Makuwa M, Telfer P, Onanga R, Dubreuil G, Chen Z, Smith SM, Georges A, Gao F, Hahn BH, and Marx PA. 1998. Natural infection of a household pet red-capped mangabey (*Cercocebus torquatus torquatus*) with a new simian immunodeficiency virus. *Journal of Virology* 72:600–608.

Hahn BH, Shaw GM, De Cock KM, and Sharp PM. 2000. AIDS as a zoonosis: Scientific and public health implications. *Science* 287:607–614.

Jin MJ, Rogers J, Phillips-Conroy JE, Allan JS, Desrosiers RC, Shaw GM, Sharp PM, and Hahn BH. 1994a. Infection of a yellow baboon with simian immunodeficiency virus from African green monkeys: Evidence for cross-species transmission in the wild. *Journal of Virology* 68:8454–8460.

Jin MJ, Hui H, Robertson DL, Müller MC, Barre-Sinoussi F, Hirsch VM, Allan JS, Shaw GM, Sharp PM, and Hahn BH. 1994b. Mosaic genome structure of simian immunodeficiency virus from west African green monkeys. *The European Molecular Biology Organization Journal* 13:2935–2947.

Kaye JA, de Mar Melero-Montes M, and Jick H. 2001. Mumps, measles, and rubella vaccine and the incidence of autism recorded by general practitioners: A time trend analysis. *British Medical Journal* 322:460–463.

Kuiken C, Foley B, Hahn BH, Marx P, McCutchan F, Mellors J, Mullins J, Wolinsky S, and Korber B. 1999. *Human Retroviruses and AIDS: A Compilation and Analysis of Nucleic Acid and Amino Acid Sequences*. Los Alamos, NM: Los Alamos National Laboratory.

Mauclere P, Loussert-Ajaka I, Damond F, Fagot P, Souquieres S, Monny Lobe M, Mbopi Keou FX, Barre-Sinoussi F, Saragosti S, Brun-Vezinet F, and Simon F. 1997. Serological and virological characterization of HIV-1 group O infection in Cameroon. *AIDS* 11:445–453.

Ochoa EG and Lago PM. 1987. Epidemiological surveillance and control of poliomyelitis in the Republic of Cuba. *Journal of Hygiene, Epidemiology, Microbiology, and Immunology* 31(4):381–389.

Peeters M, Honore C, Huet T, Bedjabaga L, Ossari S, Bussi P, Cooper RW, and Delaporte E. 1989. Isolation and partial characterization of an HIV-related virus occurring naturally in chimpanzees in Gabon. *AIDS* 3:625–630.

Peeters M, Fransen K, Delaporte E, Van den Haesevelde M, Gershy-Damet GM, Kestens L, van der Groen G, and Piot P. 1992. Isolation and characterization of a new chimpanzee lentivirus (simian immunodeficiency virus isolate cpz-ant) from a wild-captured chimpanzee. *AIDS* 6:447–451.

Peeters M, Janssens W, Fransen K, Brandful J, Heyndrickx L, Koffi K, Delaporte E, Piot P, Gershy-Damet GM, and van der Groen G. 1994. Isolation of simian immunodeficiency viruses from two sooty mangabeys in Cote d'Ivoire: virological and genetic characterization and relationship to other HIV type 2 and SIVsm/mac strains. *AIDS Research and Human Retroviruses* 10:1289–1294.

Peeters M, Pourrut X, Bibollet-Ruche F, Courgnaud V, Abela B, Mpoudi E, Hahn B, and Delaporte E. 2001. Ongoing exposure of humans to simian immunodeficiency viruses in West Central Africa poses a risk for additional zoonotic transmissions. Paper presented at 8th Conference on Retroviruses and Opportunistic Infections, Foundation for Retrovirology and Human Health, Chicago, February 4–8, 2001.

Peltola H and Heinonen OP. 1986. Frequency of true adverse reactions to measles-mumps-rubella vaccine: A double-blind, placebo-controlled trial in twins. *Lancet* 1:939–942.

Plotkin SA and Orenstein WA, eds. 1999. *Vaccines,* 3rd ed. Philadelphia: WB Saunders.

Santiago M, Rodenburg C, Mamaeva O, Kilby J, Moldoveanu Z, Fahey B, Muller M, Ayouba A, Shaw G, McClure H, Heeney J, Nerrienet E, Boesch C, Wrangham R, Gao F, and Hahn B. 2001. AIDS as a zoonosis: characterizing the primate reservoir. Paper presented at 8th Conference on Retroviruses and Opportunistic Infections, Foundation for Retrovirology and Human Health, Chicago, February 4–8, 2001.

Sharp PM, Bailes E, Chaudhuri RR, Rodenburg CM, Santiago MO, and Hahn BH. 2001. The origins of AIDS viruses: where and when? *Philosophical Transactions of the Royal Society of London, Series B* 356:867–876.

Shulman LM, Manor Y, Handsher R, Delpeyroux F, McDonough MJ, Halmut T, Silberstein I, Alfandari J, Quay J, Fisher T, Robinov J, Kew OM, Crainic R, and Mendelson E. 2000. Molecular and antigenic characterization of a highly evolved derivative of the type 2 oral poliovaccine strain isolated from sewage in Israel. *Journal of Clinical Microbiology* 38(10):3729–3734.

Simon F, Mauclere P, Roques P, Loussert-Ajaka I, Muller-Trutwin MC, Saragosti S, Georges-Courbot MC, Barre-Sinoussi F, and Brun-Vezinet F. 1998. Identification of a new human immunodeficiency virus type 1 distinct from group M and group O. *Nature Medicine* 4:1032–1037.

Souquiere S, Bibollet-Ruche F, Robertson DL, Makuwa M, Apetrei C, Onanga R, Kornfeld C, Plantier JC, Gao F, Abernethy K, White LJ, Karesh W, Telfer P, Wickings EJ, Mauclere P, Marx PA, Barre-Sinoussi F, Hahn BH, Muller-Trutwin MC, and Simon F. 2001. Wild Mandrillus sphinx are carriers of two types of lentivirus. *Journal of Virology* 75:7086–7096.

Strebel PM, Aubert-Combiescu A, Ion-Nedelcu N, Biberi-Moroeanu S, Combiescu M, Sutter RW, Kew OM, Pallansch MA, Patriarca PA, and Cochi SL. 1994. Paralytic poliomyelitis in Romania, 1984–1992. Evidence for a high risk of vaccine-associated disease and reintroduction of wild-virus infection. *American Journal of Epidemiology* 140(12):1111–1124.

Sutter RW and Prevots R. 1994. Vaccine-associated paralytic poliomyelitis among immunodeficient persons. *Infections in Medicine* 11(6):429–438.

Ukkonen P. 1996. Rubella immunity and morbidity: impact of different vaccination programs in Finland 1979–1992. *Scandinavian Journal of Infectious Diseases* 28(1):31–35.

UNAIDS (Joint United Nations Programme on HIV/AIDS). 2000. AIDS Epidemic Update: December 2000. Online. Available at www.unaids.org.

van der Loeff MFS and Aaby P. 1999. Towards a better understanding of the epidemiology of HIV-2. *AIDS* 13 Suppl A:S69–S84.

van Rensburg EJ, Engelbrecht S, Mwenda J, Laten JD, Robson BA, Stander T, and Chege GK. 1998. Simian immunodeficiency viruses (SIVs) from eastern and southern Africa: Detection of a SIVagm variant from a chacma baboon. *Journal of General Virology* 79:1809–1814.

Vidal N, Peeters M, Mulanga-Kabeya C, Nzilambi N, Robertson D, Ilunga W, Sema H, Tshimanga K, Bongo B, and Delaporte E. 2000. Unprecedented degree of human immunodeficiency virus type 1 (HIV-1) group M genetic diversity in the Democratic Republic of Congo suggests that the HIV-1 pandemic originated in central Africa. *Journal of Virology* 74:10498–10507.

Wilkie D, Shaw E, Rotberg F, Morelli G, and Auzel P. 2000. Roads, development, and conservation in the Congo Basin. *Conservation Biology* 14:1614–1622.

Yoshida H, Horie H, Matsuura K, and Miyamura T. 2000. Characterisation of vaccine-derived polioviruses isolated from sewage and river water in Japan. *Lancet* 356(9240):1461–1463.

4

Operational and Institutional Challenges to Post-Eradication

OVERVIEW

The greatest impediment to eradication is the accidental or intentional reintroduction or re-emergence of infection. Non-human reservoirs of infection, accidental reintroduction from a stasis reservoir, reversion of the vaccine strain virus to virulence, recombination between vaccine and wild-type virus, the evolution of new viruses, ecological niches left vacant after vaccination, and malevolent intent are all potential sources of reintroduction for which we need to be fully prepared.

Reintroduction could strike anywhere. Increased movement of people across international borders complicates the challenge of combating unexpected disease outbreaks and preventing global spread. Prevention of reintroduction requires detecting infection while outbreaks are still locally confined, which means that a national surveillance system supported by accurate laboratory-based diagnosis must be firmly established. In addition to serving as a regulatory framework for global surveillance, the proposed revision of the International Health Regulations (IHR) provides a functional and effective template for national surveillance in countries that do not already have an effective system in place.

One of the greatest challenges in the IHR revision process is ensuring that reporting of public health risk expands to all urgent international public health events, instead of focusing only on specific diseases. Countries and institutions need to be able to act as a network of networks in order to identify and limit the damage caused by new outbreaks, while simultaneously minimizing unnecessary overreaction, economic hardship, and social instability.

In many countries, global eradication priorities override local health priorities. In the past, this has been justified by cost-effectiveness analyses demonstrating the enormous savings expected when an infectious agent is declared eradicated. Now, however, we are beginning to realize that strengthening local health service infrastructures can operate synergistically with global priorities. Indeed, empowering communities with the resources to manage their public health problems in a self-reliant way is the best framework for dealing with disease outbreaks.

Finally, prevention of reintroduction requires the safe containment of post-eradication agents in order to protect against accidental or intentional transmission of eradicated agents. Good practices are needed for the acquisition, preservation, authentication, and distribution of infectious materials for legitimate research and clinical purposes. Heightened laboratory containment and security will be an increasingly essential part of the biological research infrastructure in the post-immunization era.

REVISION OF THE INTERNATIONAL HEALTH REGULATIONS: PROGRESS REPORT

Marlo Libel, M.D., M.P.H.

Epidemiologist, Communicable Diseases Program
Division of Disease Prevention and Control
Pan American Health Organization, Washington, D.C.

The International Health Regulations (IHR) were the first multilateral initiative for the surveillance of cross-border transmission of infectious diseases. They are currently the only binding set of regulations on global surveillance for infectious diseases by World Health Organization (WHO) member states. In response to the threat of cross-border transmission posed by substantial increases in international travel, the World Health Assembly (WHA) requested the revision of the IHR in 1995. The original public health protection measures for international travelers, conveyances, goods, and cargoes will remain in the revised IHR, but they will be subject to review and consultation.

The fundamental principle of the IHR is to ensure maximum security against international spread of disease with minimum interference with world traffic and trade. To achieve this purpose, the present IHR oblige member states to notify WHO of cholera, plague, and yellow fever outbreaks in their territories, list the maximum measures applicable during such outbreaks (based on evidence-based information), and make rules for international traffic. Listing maximum allowable measures is essential for preventing overreaction which could damage tourism, traffic, and trade and lead to unnecessarily harsh economic consequences. During the early 1990s, for example, a cholera epidemic in the Americas cost Andean countries more than $1 billion because maximum allowable measures had not been defined. These measures should be based on evidence-based information.

Although the IHR are the only international, legally binding tool for public health, they have limited use for the following reasons:

- They stipulate regulations for only three diseases (i.e., cholera, plague, and yellow fever).
- They render WHO wholly dependent upon the country suffering the outbreak to make the official notification.
- They do not provide a mechanism for collaboration between member states and WHO.
- They lack event-specific measures and incentives for compliance.

With these major constraints in mind, key changes have been proposed to develop an IHR that would adapt to emerging trends in 21st-century epidemiology and global travel.

Revised Core Concepts

Although there are some new core concepts proposed for the revised IHR, most of the changes involve developing and fine-tuning already extant rules:

Surveillance

The new IHR will neither contain a list of notifiable diseases nor depend solely on the use of syndromes for notification. Instead, they will require the reporting of all "events of urgent international importance related to public health." The reason for this is two-fold. First, in the present world of new and re-emerging diseases, any disease list could immediately become obsolete. Second, a case of a disease in and of itself does not always pose a danger of international spread or impact. The disease must be coupled to circumstances, such as place, time, size of outbreak, closeness to an international border or airport, speed of spread, mode of transmission, and so on.

Thus, routine occurrence of endemic diseases will not be notifiable under the revised IHR, and countries will not be able to send off reports about diagnosed cases in an automatic fashion. When there is an event with possible international consequences, the national administration must quickly decide if the event fulfills the WHO criteria and should be reported to WHO. The new IHR will contain a test to help administrators decide if an event is both urgent *and* international. An early draft of the algorithm, which was tested during the Syndrome Pilot Study, contained the following parameters:

- High potential for spread outside the community/country,
- Unexpectedly high case fatality ratio,
- Unusual or unexpected event,
- Country capacity to control and contain the event,
- High international media profile,
- Potential for imposition of trade/traffic barriers by other countries,
- Occurring in a high-density/urban area,
- Significant possibility of international transport of infected persons or contaminated goods/conveyances, and
- Significant possibility of vector transport.

Communication

Because the new IHR will cover a much wider span of public health events and outbreaks, and because these events may happen very quickly, 24-hour communication with WHO is critical. Information may need to be distributed nationally to hospitals, health officials, ports, and airports very quickly. Each member state should have a single, focal e-mail address that leads to someone who is available at all times. This requires a reliable electronic communication and back-up system within each member state.

Reporting Capacity

In order to ensure the quick dissemination of information regarding urgent national events of potential international importance, each country must have the capacity to quickly report, analyze, and determine the potential effect of national disease events on other member states. This will require surveillance systems that allow for rapid analysis and transfer of information on unusual and unexpected events from the periphery to the center.

The revised IHR will contain a recommended template for core requirements for a national surveillance system. In many countries, this surveillance/analysis capacity may already be in place. Others may need a grace period to fulfill this IHR requirement, and external assistance and funding may be necessary; the template could be used for defining core surveillance needs to national health sectors and external donors.

Notification

Member states will have the option to make confidential, provisional notifications to WHO. Currently, the IHR automatically lists notified cases in the *Weekly Epidemiological Record* (WER). However, in the early days of an event, it is often unclear if the criteria for an urgent international event are fulfilled. With this proposed change, member states will have the option to contact WHO on a provisional basis before any information is made public. The member state and WHO can work together to assess the extent and potential impact of the event and issue a joint statement. By collaborating with WHO before making a statement, the member state would gain credibility and reduce the likelihood of overreaction.

Information

Other information in addition to official notifications will be used by WHO to help identify and control urgent international events, and member states will respond to requests from WHO to verify the reliability of this information. Urgent international events often reach the global information super-highway and become news even before the most efficient administration has had time to react to the events and make any sort of official notification. To prevent threatened countries from responding to unverified news by restricting cross-border traffic and trade, WHO will need to inform member states and issue recommendations on appropriate measures.

Economic Considerations

In order for a global surveillance system to function well, the economic consequences of reporting disease events must be considered. If the WHO notification and response system cannot help to reduce tourism and trade losses to what is strictly required from a public health perspective, compliance with IHR reporting and notification obligations will likely be ignored by member states. Thus, the new IHR will establish a template for measures to protect other member states from unnecessary economic losses. These measures will be based on the actual public health threat or impact of the event, as determined by all available evidence. Establishing these guidelines will require input from all WHO departments involved in goods, such as Food Safety, Environment, Pharmaceuticals, as well as a plethora of external stakeholders.

Assistance

Many countries may need external assistance after provisional notification or a request from WHO for further information. Under the new guidelines, WHO will be obligated to assist member states in rapidly assessing and controlling outbreaks. If the extent and potential threat of the outbreak is unclear, WHO will offer to send a response team to collaborate with the member state government in controlling disease spread and minimizing economic damage.

By working with WHO, the affected country would receive international recognition for its effort to prevent international spread, which should reduce unnecessary economic hardship. The capacity of WHO to react and assist in outbreaks, even when there are multiple outbreaks occurring simultaneously, must be improved.

Recommendations

A transparent, decision-making process will be established within WHO to issue recommendations for member state action in case of imminent risk of international disease spread. These recommendations could be directed either at the affected country, at all other member states, or both. This will require a quick gathering of wide, representative consensus.

Preventive Measures

Just as it is impossible to list diseases, there is no way to describe appropriate measures for each event in advance. However, the revised IHR will contain a list of all key measures that could potentially be used in a WHO recommendation to prevent international disease spread at embarkation, during travel, and at point of entry. Some examples of measures potentially applicable at point of entry into non-affected member states from an affected member state are shown in Table 4-1.

During an urgent health event, WHO would use appropriate measures from the complete list as a basis for a recommendation to member states. The recommendation would be time-limited for the event, so a clear protocol for ending the measures would need to be included. To create the flexibility required to adapt to each major international threat, non-binding recommendations will have to replace the fixed, binding measures in the current IHR.

Review Process

A permanent IHR review body will be established in order to build continuity within the IHR process. Lack of a mandatory review process has rendered the existing IHR out-of-date. Plus, the new IHR will have much broader provisions and will require continuous interpretation and precedents setting.

TABLE 4-1 Measures Potentially Applicable at Point of Entry into Non-affected Member States from an Affected Member State

Travelers	Goods and Conveyances
-require travel history in affected country -require proof of medical examination -require medical examination on entry -require proof of vaccination or prophylaxis -require vaccination or other prophylaxis for entry -require protective measures for suspected cases -active or passive medical surveillance if travel from affected area -isolation of traveler for incubation period of disease -refuse entry of persons from affected area	-require inspection of conveyance, cargo, or goods -require treatment of conveyance, cargo, or goods -require isolation of conveyance, cargo, or goods -require destruction of cargo or goods -refuse entry of conveyance, cargo, or goods

The Role of WHO

The new IHR will provide global regulatory guidelines for how to respond to international disease threats, the implementation of which WHO will coordinate. Even though the best way to prevent international spread of disease is to detect public health threats early and stamp them out when they are still a small, local problem, national efforts often require international coordination. Many countries need assistance from multilateral institutions for their national surveillance systems. Plus, even localized national events can quickly affect international traffic. Thus, an international coordinator is critical for standardizing notifications, responses from other countries, and the global exchange of epidemiological information. Effective notification of disease events to WHO will be facilitated by an assurance of how this information will affect member states' economic interests. All of the various functions that WHO would serve as international coordinator in response to a disease event are included in Figure 4-1.

IHR Benefits to Member States

The new IHR will benefit member states in a variety of ways:

- National surveillance systems will need to be improved.
- Modern communication systems for detecting and responding to

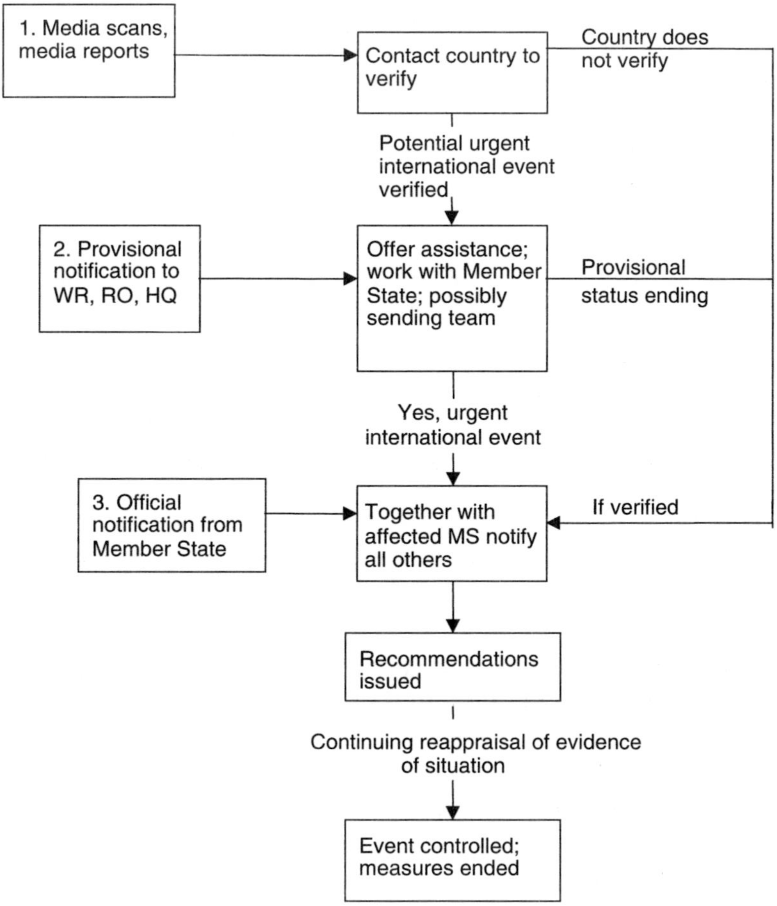

FIGURE 4-1 Possible framework for IHR response. SOURCE: PAHO/WHO.

potential international health events will need to be developed in countries where they are not already available.

- Disturbances to free traffic, which constitute an obstacle to reporting, will need to be thwarted.
- A set of generic rules to handle different kinds of urgent events and a rapid mechanism to agree on appropriate levels of national protection within this set of rules will be developed by the IHR for implementation in member countries.

Ideally, the IHR revision process should involve broad consensus with all member states. The current collaboration between the Secretariat and interested member states is designed to test proposed changes and seek suggestions on how the member states want the new IHR to operate. An electronic virtual discussion forum has been set up between the IHR team and representatives of WHO member states, and the revision team has written to all member states asking them to nominate individuals who will provide input to the revision process. In Latin America, the Pan American Health Organization (PAHO) has been working with Mexico, Peru, Brazil, and signatory states of the Mercado Común del Sur (MERCOSUR) to establish formal collaboration partnerships for the IHR revision process, and MERCOSUR has listed IHR revision follow-up as an agenda topic for its health sector committee.

The next stage of consensus-building involves steering working relationships among WHO country representatives, member states, WHO regional offices, and international agencies and institutions whose work is related to the IHR. These international agencies include the Food and Agriculture Organization (FAO), International Air and Transport Association (IATA), International Civil Aviation Organization (ICAO), World Trade Organization (WTO), and International Maritime Organization (IMO).

DISEASE SURVEILLANCE, PROGRAM MANAGEMENT, AND SUSTAINMENT OF IMMUNIZATION PROGRAMS

Donald S. Burke, M.D.

Professor of International Health
Director, Center for Immunization Research
Johns Hopkins School of Hygiene and Public Health, Baltimore, MD

A major challenge to post-eradication is knowing how long disease surveillance should be continued, both during immunization and after it. Surveillance is also an important control issue for other viral diseases, such as yellow fever, that are not currently slated for eradication but for which vaccines are available and in various stages of implementation worldwide.

Following is a review of several disease control programs and lessons to be learned from their historical examples.

Polio Surveillance and Program Management

Laboratory surveillance has been crucial to the success of the polio eradication campaigns. Surveillance measures include:

- detection and reporting of all cases of acute flaccid paralysis (AFP),

- collection of two stool specimens within the first 14 days after the onset of paralysis,
- isolation and characterization of enteroviruses in cell cultures with particular attention to the polioviruses, and
- differentiation between the wild type and polio vaccine virus strains.

Differentiating the oral polio vaccine strains is a major challenge to laboratory surveillance because it requires a relatively cumbersome cell culture technique. This is true despite a global network of functional polio eradication laboratories; most small country laboratories experience difficulties performing the specialized technique.

An example of a typical surveillance caseload is Mongolia, where there are about 1,000 reporting districts throughout the country that participate in ongoing surveillance. Over the past three years, these reporting districts have detected 90 cases of AFP. All 80% of the cases for which specimens were available for laboratory differentiation were confirmed not to be polio. The other 20%, for which specimens were unavailable or inadequate for laboratory analysis, were confirmed not to be polio based on clinical evaluation: either there was no residual paralysis on long-term follow-up or, if there was, expert clinical review of the case confirmed that it was not polio. The last confirmed case of polio in Mongolia was in 1993.

Measles Surveillance and Program Management

Measles cases can be mistaken for dengue, rubella, scarlet fever, and roseola, the clinical manifestations of which overlap and make differential diagnosis difficult. Consequently, as for polio, laboratory surveillance for measles is very important, especially if eradication requires detecting and reporting all compatible cases.

In contrast to polio, measles diagnosis is made by detection of IgM antibodies, not virus isolation. Measles infection usually occurs 14 days before the onset of rash, and anti-measles IgM typically appears within the first few days after the rash. The sensitivity of the IgM assay in the first few days after rash is 60 or 70%, and nearly 100% by the fourth day. Diagnostic accuracy relies on the proper timing of specimen collection.

As with polio, routine diagnosis is usually done in one of the many eradication network laboratories currently being developed worldwide.

Lessons from Yellow Fever Program Management

The first attempts at yellow fever eradication were the early campaigns sponsored by the Rockefeller Foundation. In 1915, Wickliffe Rose, the Director of the International Health Commission of the Rockefeller Foundation, said that the "international commission was prepared to give aid to eradication of this disease in those areas where the infection is endemic and where conditions would seem to invite cooperation for its control."

One of the major reasons these early yellow fever eradication efforts failed was the presence of jungle yellow fever: a cycle of disease that existed in non-human primates and was transmitted by vectors other than *Aedes aegypti*. During his investigations of epidemics near Muzo, Columbia, in 1907, Colombian scientist Dr. Franco made several observations that led him to believe that jungle yellow fever existed: the disease could be contracted in the forest as well as urban neighborhoods; it was transmitted by other culicine vectors in addition to *Ae. aegypti*; and its transmission occurred during daylight hours.

After the 1915 declaration to eradicate yellow fever, William Crawford Gorgas—famous for eradicating yellow fever from Cuba and the Panama Canal Zone—led a commission into Muzo, Colombia, to investigate reports of yellow fever. The existence of jungle yellow fever was not recognized at the time, and the commission believed that *Ae. aegypti* had to be present in order for yellow fever to be transmitted. So when they found no evidence of *Ae. aegypti*, they concluded that the reported disease could not be yellow fever. Thus, the eradication campaign proceeded in the face of what was most certainly unrecognized jungle yellow fever. It was not until 1935 that Dr. Fred Soper, Regional Director of the Rockefeller Foundation's International Health Division in Rio de Janeiro, acknowledged Franco's contribution and finally agreed that jungle yellow fever existed.

The Rockefeller yellow fever program extended into Africa as well, where a yellow fever research laboratory was built in Entebbe, Uganda, in 1936. Although its primary focus initially was yellow fever, over the years this laboratory has been involved with a variety of other viral diseases as well. For example, the West Nile virus was first isolated there in 1938, and studies conducted at the laboratory in the 1930s provided an early understanding of the ecology and epidemiology of this virus. The facility now houses a major AIDS laboratory, as well as polio and measles surveillance laboratories. Thus, the initial yellow fever investment has resulted in a number of positive spin-offs.

The lessons to be learned from yellow fever eradication and control initiatives are, first, that field research is essential to making sound policy decisions. We need to beware of false epidemiological dogma. Second, even a "failed" program can leave a strong legacy on which to build.

Influenza

Although influenza has never been eradicated, major variants of influenza virus, such as H1N1, have spontaneously disappeared. By using

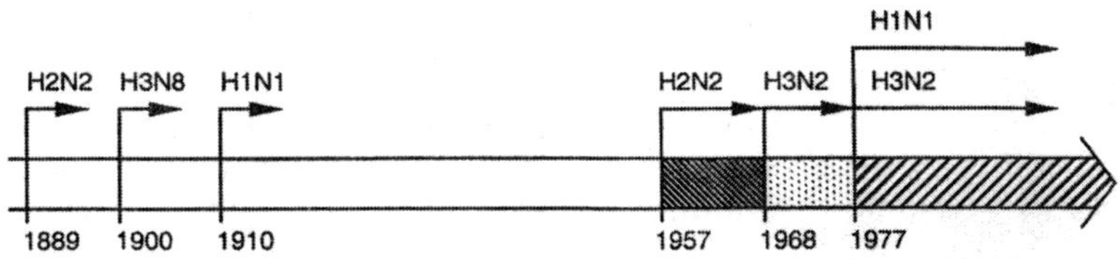

FIGURE 4-2 Sero-archeology: Recycling of influenza A viruses in humans?

seroarcheology to examine past cohorts of infected persons, it is possible to reconstruct the major epidemics of influenza by their hemagglutinin and neuraminidase types.

H1N1s dominated the global circulation of influenza virus until the 1950s, when it disappeared and was replaced by H2N2 and H3N2 strains. In 1977, H1N1 surprisingly reappeared (Figure 4-2). Research on viral genomics strongly suggests that the reappearance of the H1N1 Russian 1977 influenza probably originated from a laboratory stock culture. H1N1 first re-appeared in Anshan in northern China in May 1977, and then spread worldwide. The gene sequence of the 1977 H1N1 strain is essentially identical to the gene sequence of the 1950 strain of H1N1, suggesting that the virus was probably in frozen stasis during its inter-epidemic years. Its re-emergence occurred slightly after the U.S. swine flu scare; the virus was probably taken out of the freezer in response to concerns about spreads of H1 and N1 viruses. The lesson to be learned from the re-emergence of H1N1 is that *accidental reintroduction is a real threat.*

Smallpox

Smallpox has been covered in great detail elsewhere in this report. However, a major point to re-emphasize is the newly learned lesson that reintroduction of viruses through *human malice is a serious threat.*

Adenoviruses

Adenoviruses are the best example of an *evolving or re-emerging virus that is filling an ecological niche left vacant after vaccination.* Adeno-viruses, particularly types 4 and 7, are a major problem in military populations. The adenovirus vaccines were developed and clinically tested in the late 1960s and early 1970s. Data suggest that the use of the adeno 4 vaccine led to an absolute increase in the incidence of adeno 7 infections. For example, at one post at Fort Lewis, what was initially an adeno 4 epidemic evolved into an adeno 7 epidemic after 10 weeks of using the adeno 4 vaccine, suggesting that adeno 7 had moved into a vacant niche previously occupied by adeno 4.

These findings may have relevance for other immunization programs, such as polio. For example, sequence analysis of the RNA polymerase of the enteroviruses shows that the phylogenies of the Coxsackie A viruses and the polioviruses are intertwined. It has been hypothesized that the only difference between these viruses is the host recognition receptor: polioviruses use the CD155, and the Coxsackie viruses use the ICAM 1. It is possible that a simple receptor switch would provide variants of Coxsackie viruses with properties more like polioviruses. The question is, will Coxsackie A viruses fill the vacated poliovirus niche?

Polioviruses

Detailed discussion about polio revertants and recombinants is provided elsewhere in this report. For example, known instances of reversions of polio vaccines, including the Poland USOL and several Sabin strains, that have led to vaccine-associated paralytic polio (VAPP) epidemics are presented in Table 4-2. Also, a natural recombinant polio wild type Sabin-1 circulated in China for several years; and toward the end of the polio epidemic and the eradication of polio in China, a recombinant strain containing sequences from the Sabin vaccine strain spread from person to person, infecting thousands of Chinese. Early lessons learned from the poliovirus are that *viral evolvability can introduce unexpected wild cards.*

Viral evolvability raises concerns about all forms of live attenuated vaccines with a proven capacity to efficiently swap genes between humans and animals. Of particular concern are live attenuated vaccines with segmented genomes, such as influenza and rotavirus, for which we can almost certainly expect recombinant variants of wild type and vaccine type to emerge. Hopefully, none will be more virulent or more transmissible than the wild type parent.

TABLE 4-2 Reversion of Polio Vaccine to Virulence with Epidemic Spread

Year	Country	Virus (Vaccine)	# Cases
1968	Poland	Polio-3 (USOL)	464
1988–1993	Egypt	Polio-2 (Sabin)	32
Mid-1990s	China	Polio-2 (Sabin)	NR
Late-1990s	Israel	Polio-2 (Sabin)	(0)
2000	Dominican Republic/Haiti	Polio-1 (Sabin)	19

Hepatitis B Virus

All current hepatitis B virus (HBV) vaccines are either inactivated or not capable of replication. Immunity is directed largely against a particular immunodominant hydrophilic loop of the surface antigen of hepatitis B. In many immunized persons, the loop has significant amino acid substitutions that substantially change immunogenicity. These variants are the predominant type of virus present in as many as 20–30% of vaccinees who become infected. Long-term models predict that it will take 30 or 40 years for these escape variants to predominate worldwide. The early lesson learned from HBV is that *virus variants may emerge, particularly for vaccines targeting a single major epitope.* Virus variants of live attenuated vaccines or complex antigens are less likely to emerge.

Conclusion

Several lessons can be learned from our past efforts to control or eradicate viral diseases:

- Yellow fever: The presence of a non-human reservoir (i.e., jungle yellow fever) creates the likelihood for continued reintroduction.
- Influenza: Accidental reintroduction can result from a stasis reservoir.
- Smallpox: Malevolent reintroduction poses a serious threat.
- Polio: A vaccine strain can revert to virulence and/or recombination between vaccine and natural virus.
- Hepatitis B: "Immune escape" mutants of wild-type virus can evolve and eventually predominate worldwide.
- HIV: Natural viruses are actively emerging (see Chapter 2).

Francois-Joseph Broussais (1772–1839), one of Napoleon's personal physicians, referred to the "genius of the epidemic." Given the already proven cleverness of the viruses in their ability to frustrate our immunization strategies, we should carefully consider how viruses might thwart our eradication efforts and how we can detect and promptly counter those moves.

Surveillance is crucial to successful eradication. As eradication campaigns near completion, the potential for viral surprises will increase, not decrease. "Forward" laboratories are a vital part of surveillance. Laboratory capacity should be strengthened, especially in regions where eradication is difficult and/or variants are likely to emerge.

THE CAPACITY OF PUBLIC HEALTH SERVICES TO RESPOND TO AN OUTBREAK IN THE POST-ERADICATION ERA

Carl E. Taylor, M.D., M.P.H.

Professor Emeritus, Department of International Health
Johns Hopkins School of Hygiene and Public Health, Baltimore, MD

During global eradication initiatives, global priorities tend to override local priorities. Evidence suggests, however, that there are cost-effective, synergistic ways to meet both objectives simultaneously. Indeed, empowering local communities with strong primary health care infrastructures which they can rely on to solve their own problems is the best way to prevent emerging disease outbreaks. New advances in Community-Based Primary Health Care (CBPHC) provide new hope for building synergisms between competing goals in order to cope with emerging infections.

In accordance with the World Health Assembly resolution in 1988, nations made a commitment to pursue polio eradication "in ways which strengthen the development of immunization programmes as a whole, fostering its contribution, in turn, to the development of the health infrastructure and of primary health care." Recently, this level of commitment has been evaluated in several ways.

Recent Reports

A 1993 PAHO commission involving a detailed qualitative assessment of polio eradication (PE) in six Latin American countries concluded that PE strengthened health systems in countries that already had a basic health infrastructure. This success could not, however, be extrapolated to countries with weak health systems. The greatest positive impact of PE was on social mobilization and intersectoral cooperation, two of the three main goals of the Alma Ata World Conference on Primary Health Care in 1978. However, negative effects were also seen, mainly competition between components of the health infrastructure as a result of aggressive targeting.

Other recent evaluations of the great progress in worldwide PE call for a greater awareness of the fact that the eradication experience will be different in places where health services are weak or nonexistent compared to places with well-established health systems, as was shown in malaria eradication efforts in the 1960s.

Comprehensive recommendations have been made about the many "missed opportunities" and the need for a new organizational framework to strengthen the health service infrastructure. Recommendations from a WHO meeting in December 1999 include:

- Monitor "key indicators" of impact on health systems.
- Compile existing documentation, especially gaps in equity, community ownership, political will, public-private partnership, peace building, Vitamin A supplements, laboratory capacity, and opportunity costs.
- Establish an oversight committee for the health systems-strengthening aspect of the PE goal.
- Engage broader participation of those with expertise in health systems to ensure action on "missed opportunities."

The WHO report warned that "as polio eradication enters its most difficult stages, many health experts express their concerns that the WHA promise ... will not be achieved, unless greater efforts are made. Intensive, accelerated, polio activities are underway ... and the fear, expressed by some, is that there will not be enough staff time or energy to take on the broader agenda of strengthening routine immunization and health systems. . . . Today, routine immunization coverage is at the lowest it has been in a decade in many countries and health systems have not effectively responded to decentralization, particularly in the provision of preventive services." Finally, the report suggests that help will be needed from GAVI (Global Alliance for Vaccines and Immunization), presumably because the amount of money needed has dramatically increased.

Dilemma

In the past, the costs of focusing only on direct eradication services have been justified by cost-effectiveness calculations indicating that when PE is declared there will be a savings of at least $1.5 billion per year per country. Thus, countries where wild virus still occurs are pressured to pay more attention to the global priority for PE rather than the diseases killing their own children. Now, however, we are beginning to realize the importance of strengthening local health systems.

Deficiencies in diagnostic and treatment capacity decrease surveillance capacity and can create a long time lag between the occurrence and identification of outbreaks. Identification of outbreaks will be especially important after eradication is declared complete, and it is critical that local health systems be strengthened in order to meet this demand. Stronger local health systems are also needed to increase child immunization rates.

UNICEF is now using independent surveys for the State of the World's Children Report and is changing some of its earlier claims about child immunization patterns of the past decade. In India, between 1999 and 2000, the percentage of children reported as fully immunized dropped on average 20 points, from the 80s to the 60s. In China, at the same time, immunization rates dropped on average 10 percentage points.

There are tremendous differences in immunization rates within countries, as shown by data from the USAID-funded Demographic and Health Surveys in India. The Pulse Polio National Immunization Days (NIDs) that began in 1995 have resulted in the greatest public health events in history with reports of having reached more than 100 million children. Rates in the advanced southwestern states of India were already good, and the NIDs raised them to over 90%. However, in the north central states of India where the rates were low, they remain low. Twenty-nine percent of children in two Indian north central states (Uttar Pradesh and Arunachal Pradesh) still had no reported immunizations. Uttar Pradesh's population is equivalent to the 10th largest country in the world. Similar reports are emerging from Africa.

Need for Cooperation for Adequate Surveillance

There is abundant evidence that PE efforts and actions to strengthen local health systems can produce powerful synergisms. PE depends on both NIDs and surveillance, both of which in turn depend on technological mobilization and research on the changing nature of health services. They also depend on flexible methods of social mobilization to bring vaccines and children together and ways to identify and diagnose acute flaccid paralysis (AFP). The technological mobilization is straightforward, especially when outside funding for campaigns is available. However, the reality is that equipment lasts only about 10 years in developing countries and vaccines have to be paid for annually.

There is great uncertainty about the sustainability of social mobilization. In the past, social mobilization has been based on a passive and unsustainable model. However, there is an alternative model which relies on community empowerment that works amazingly rapidly if programs are organized to promote community self-reliance rather than dependency. In recent years, there has been great progress in understanding the process of community empowerment. It is no longer necessary to assume, as we did earlier, that community empowerment happens by chance.

It has, for many of us, been baffling and contrary to other experience to see the success of social mobilization for polio. Everyone, and especially the bureaucrats doing the implementation, have been amazed at the response. Even the poorest countries can generate a local commitment that brings together immunizations and mothers and children in the most massive health events of all time. Global pressure has made leaders of the poorest countries feel ashamed if they do not cooperate and mobilize all government resources for this global priority. The local commitment was understandable for vaccine campaigns targeted at one of the main causes of child death. But it is unclear why the commmitment persists for a disease that is so rare that local peoples have no name for it and, in some places, efforts to educate the people about the disease involve searching for relatively rare cases with residual paralysis to use as audiovisual aids. Why do the local people think that there is so much official concern for these diseases? Do they think that the vaccinations have some special power? Do they think the oral drops will make it less necessary for their children to receive the painful injections that make them cry? How long will poor countries continue to let global priorities completely override local priorities? And, most importantly, what can we do so that the remarkable public enthusiasm for PE social mobilization enhances other immunization programs and promotes interventions for the main infections that cause death in each locality, thereby truly balancing global and local priorities?

Although the amazing and highly publicized advances in technical and social mobilization for PE are impressive, there have also been parallel but not publicized advances in community-based primary health care. It is time to bring the two streams of progress together. Evidence shows that building primary health care infrastructure is not necessarily expensive and slow. After the Alma Ata Conference, the claim was made by donors that comprehensive primary health care does not go to scale and only selective approaches can be extended. However, we now know that sustainable services can be expanded remarkably rapidly to cover whole regions.

The key issue is whether the social mobilization necessary for NIDs and surveillance can be accomplished using an approach that will not collapse when outside funding and expatriates are gone. Great effort is already being directed toward building capacity and mobilizing volunteers, so it will only take a little more patience to build a self-reliant community. Top-down processes create dependency, not self-reliance.

A remarkable feature of the new process is that it includes the best hope for long term financing. International Monetary Fund (IMF) economic reforms cut health budgets in Africa by a third to a half in the 1980s. Donors dumped responsibility for public health back onto countries, except for the few diseases that could be attacked by campaigns, and countries dumped responsibility onto communities. It is clear that communities will eventually have to assume responsibility for self-financing, except for the very poor who will need subsidization and for whom sustainable financing must be found. Talk about insurance is relevant only for people with resources. Now, with worldwide privatization of health care and pharmaceuticals, the prospects for care for the poor seem even more jeopardized unless international equity is taken seriously.

Conclusion

Objective research is needed to determine if scientific and technical improvements in immunization strategies better control infectious diseases. Research is also needed to gain a better understanding of the role of social mobilization in successful immunization programs. How can this amazing phenomenon be used to build a sustainable local capacity for solving a nation's own public health problems? Strong local health services and empowered communities are the best framework for preventing the disease outbreaks that this conference is addressing.

LABORATORY SECURITY AND REGULATIONS GOVERNING VIRAL PATHOGENS IN A POST-IMMUNIZATION ERA

Raymond H. Cypess, D.V.M., Ph.D., President and CEO

Frank P. Simione, M.S., Vice President, Safety and Regulatory Affairs

American Type Culture Collection (ATCC), Manassas, VA

Managing virus stocks under good laboratory security and in compliance with current regulations can best be accomplished by applying practices currently in place at Biological Resource Centers (BRCs) (Table 4-3). BRCs play an essential role in the biological research infrastructure by coordinating the shared use of validated biomaterial and data among government agencies, industry, academia, and the public. They serve as repositories, service providers, and knowledge managers. They authenticate, preserve, and distribute living cells, genomes, model organisms, research tools, and information relating to heredity and functions of living systems.

Of particular relevance to public health and infectious disease programs are BRCs that specialize in microbiology. These are collections of culturable organisms, viable but not yet culturable organisms, replicable parts of these materials, and associated data. BRCs relieve storage and distribution burdens for investigators and institutions, and they provide controlled on-site biosecurity and access to their holdings. Types of BRCs include:[1]

---

[1]Key to abbreviations: ATCC, American Type Culture Collection; BDSC, Bloomington Drosophila Stock Center, Indiana University; CBS, Centraalbureau voor Schimmelcultures; CDC, Centers for Disease Control and Prevention; CGC, Caenorhabditis Genetics Center; Coriell Institute for Medical Research, New Jersey; DSMZ, Deutsche Sammlung von Mikroorganismen und Zellkulturen GmbH; IFO, Institute for Fermentation, Osaka; JCM, Japan Collection of Microorganisms; NRCC, National Resource Center for Cephalopods, University of Texas; RPRC, Regional Primate Research Center; RSMAS, Rosenstiel School of Marine and Atmospheric Science; USDA, U.S. Department of Agriculture

- Microorganisms (e.g., ATCC, CBS, CDC, DSMZ, JCM),
- Plant germplasm, i.e., seeds, clones, cells, and tissue (e.g., ATCC, DSMZ, USDA),
- Animal cells and tissue (e.g., ATCC, Coriell, IFO),
- Vertebrate models (e.g., rodents at Jackson Laboratories, primates at RPRC, zebrafish at University of Oregon), and
- Invertebrate models (e.g., *Drosophila* at BDSC, nematodes at CGC, *Aplysia* at RSMAS, cephalopods at NRCC).

A challenge to eradication is identifying where viral stocks are currently housed, which requires a systematic inventory of existing biorepository holdings. Persons responsible for the materials must be forthcoming in complying with requests for this information.

As laboratories are identified, an attempt should be made to transfer all specimens to those biorepositories that demonstrate well-developed and documented procedures for safe handling and security. Good biorepository management practice requires documenting, managing and securing strain data, ensuring safe handling in the laboratory and in the biorepository, and strict management of access to and distribution of the agent.

Storage in select biorepository holdings will ensure that the agents are available for ongoing laboratory studies, as needed, with minimal risk of reintroducing the disease into the general population and environment. Agents that present a grave danger to a post-immunization community

TABLE 4-3 The Role of Biological Resource Centers

- Provide central source and controlled access to standard biomaterials, reagents, and data
- Provide controlled conditions for on-site biosecurity
- Provide central source of technical support
- Minimize redundancy of biomaterials
- Relieve storage and distribution burdens for investigators
- Coordinate regulatory compliance
- Provide safety deposit for essential germplasm
- Support equitable sharing of biomaterials
- Provide intellectual property management and services
- Provide knowledge management and distribution
- Promote translation of research discoveries into practical applications
- Facilitate industrialization of technologies in medicine, public health, pharmacy, agriculture, food, and environment

should be stored in facilities with Biosafety Level 4 (BSL-4) containment capability.

Admittance to material can be restricted by providing secure, controlled access to the viral agents. Levels of access should be established so that the most dangerous strains have the greatest restrictions for access and use. End-users should be qualified to work with the agent, and their institutions capable of ensuring adequate biocontainment and security.

BRC Lab Security

Acceptable acquisition practices start with a sound demonstrated knowledge of the material and its potential hazards. Acquisition is usually accompanied by material acquisition agreements which can be used to record information on the agent, its potential laboratory risk, and conditions under which the material is being provided to the biorepository. In order to ensure that the agent is safely and securely maintained in a viable unchanged state, low-temperature storage with redundant controls on equipment should be used to maintain cryopreserved stocks, and multi-response alarm monitoring should be available.

All work performed on the virus stocks in the laboratory must be conducted under good biosafety practices. Potential hazards should be identified through risk assessments and, where appropriate, laboratory workers should be immunized. However, live viral vaccines such as those available for poliovirus may present a risk if immunized laboratory staff shed the virus outside the laboratory and potentially expose a non-immunized community. Those agents posing serious risk to the community should be handled under BSL-3 containment and practices, and some agents may require BSL-4 containment.

Disposal must avoid risks associated with handling of infectious materials. The best practice is inactivation of biological materials in the laboratory, as required for BSL-3 and BSL-4 containment. Even in a BSL-2 laboratory, accommodations should be made for destruction of biohazardous agents within the laboratory area.

Internal security is especially important for stocks that cause disease for which immunization has been discontinued or that create a high risk of life-threatening disease. Physical access to the virus stocks can be controlled by securing freezers with combination or key locks that require two people to unlock the freezer and by controlling access to the area of the facility where the freezers are housed. Physical access to the biorepository can also be controlled by using key-card or other individual access identifiers. Additional safeguards include denying individuals access to both the biorepository and freezer, thus requiring two people to obtain or deposit biohazardous agents.

Freezer inventories should be designed so that a locator code is needed to find the desired material. Locator codes can be kept in strictly controlled, secure databases. Access to freezers would be denied to those who also have access to the locator codes, again requiring two people to retrieve or deposit material. Chain of custody documentation—a system of sign-offs that tracks the movement of materials—should be established to verify authorized access to the material. Evidence of the disposition of all material released to a laboratory, including destruction of records, should also be documented.

Access and Transfer of BRC Materials to Outside Sources

A mechanism for verifying a recipient's legitimate need for the material must be established and controlled independently of the biorepository. The recipient should be located at an institution where work with the agent is approved and all necessary safety and security policies and practices are in place. A mechanism such as that used by the Centers for Disease Control and Prevention (CDC) for controlling the transfer of designated select agents should be used for agents for which immunization has ceased (*Code of Federal Regulations* 42, Part 72.6).

The greatest risk of transferring viral agents to an outside laboratory is the potential for an unqualified end-user to gain access to the virus. Therefore, there must be some way to ensure that the receiving laboratory is capable of controlling access and preventing the release of restricted etiological agents to known or suspected persons, institutions, or countries that represent a proliferation risk for biowarfare or bioterrorism. With the aid of appropriate federal authorities, including the departments of Commerce, State, and Treasury, the biorepository must be able to screen potential recipients.

Distribution of disease-causing viral agents requires strict adherence to the permit and licensing requirements of local, state, federal, and international agencies. End-users should process requests for their material through an institutionally controlled system that identifies materials needing special permits and licenses. The biorepository should be familiar with the regulations on packaging, shipping, and tracking to ensure safe and controlled transfer of material.

For example, the release of any biological material from ATCC—regardless of risk category—requires that the requestor provide an organizational profile and documented assurance that the facility is equipped to handle the material safely and securely. In addition, all requests for biological materials from ATCC are screened against U.S. government lists of denied individuals, entities, and embargoed countries, and all required permits and licenses are applied where appropriate.

Conclusion

Assuring the security of post-eradication viral agents is critical to successful eradication. But it is only achievable if good practices for the acquisition, preservation, authentication, and distribution of the materials are applied. BRCs can continue to provide safe and secure management and control stocks of post-eradication viral agents. It is critical, however, that access to potentially dangerous microbial agents be controlled under strict guidelines and regulations mandated outside the BRCs, and that BRCs function solely as a means of ensuring compliance with these requirements.

5

Medical Intervention and Technological Solutions

OVERVIEW

The post-eradication era is a period of history for which there has been no precedent whatsoever in terms of a zero base of immunity. Cessation of immunization will eventually create a population susceptible to widespread infection in the event of accidental or intentional reintroduction or re-emergence of the eradicated virus. Thus, even after immunization ceases, vaccine production must continue.

However, many currently available vaccines may not be appropriate for continued post-eradication vaccine production or reinstatement. Vaccines must be continually improved and ongoing vaccination research maintained. Other potentially useful antiviral strategies—antivirals, prophylaxis, and probiotics—must also be considered as means to strengthen the immune system and serve as adjuvant or prophylactic therapies.

In the case of polio, for example, it remains to be determined which vaccine (oral polio vaccine [OPV] or inactivated polio vaccine [IPV]), or variant thereof, should be produced in the post-eradication, post-vaccination era. A detailed plan for vaccine production will require more information on OPV-derived viral persistence and transmission, as well as continuing dialogue between public health and research communities in order to ensure that appropriate vaccination research continues.

The immune system may face unforeseeable challenges when immunity in the community at large wanes in the post-immunization era, and even immunized individuals may be at risk. Molecular biology technology has advanced to the point where antiviral drugs could be developed to target specific viruses. With the exception of HIV and influenza, however, diseases for which antiviral therapy has been considered are not usually considered epidemic. The research community and pharmaceutical industry must make a concerted commitment to developing antiviral therapies for use as potential adjuvants for vaccine-preventable diseases.

Immunoprophylaxis includes both nonspecific approaches to stimulation of innate antiviral defenses and specific prophylaxis directed at particular pathogens. Currently, the best understood nonspecific prophylaxis is interferon (IFN) α/β. However, viruses display tremendous variability in their reponses to the effects of IFN α/β, and many viruses have evolved ways around IFN α/β's antiviral pathways. As is the case for antivirals, technology has advanced to a point where specific prophylactics could be developed for use against vaccine-preventable diseases—including smallpox, polio, and measles—but this has not been done.

Finally, current studies suggest that probiotic bacteria—living microbes introduced into the body in order to improve intestinal microbial balance—could be used to strengthen the immune system, even in immuncompromised individuals. Novel microbial mechanisms need to be further studied for their potential use as antigen delivery vehicles and adjuvants.

In an age of unprecedented successful vaccination initiatives, public and private sector support has led to the rapid development of vaccines for numerous infectious diseases. Implementation of these products has helped encourage confidence in the biomedical research and public health communities and garnered political will for disease eradication initiatives. This support, confidence, and political will must continue in the post-eradication era. Strong commitment is needed from both the public and private sectors to share the costs and risks associated with developing new vaccines and therapeutic products which may have only a very short product life cycle. Effective and appropriate antiviral therapies are critical for the protection of future populations in a post-immunization era.

THE POLIO ERADICATION EFFORT: SHOULD VACCINE ERADICATION BE NEXT?

Vincent R. Racaniello, Ph.D.

Higgins Professor, Department of Microbiology
Columbia University College of Physicians and Surgeons
New York, NY

The World Health Organization (WHO) goal to eradicate polio by the year 2000 (now extended to 2005) has resulted in an extraordinary reduction in global incidence of the disease. According to the WHO global plan, vaccination can stop when eradication is certified, laboratory stocks of poliovirus are contained, and there is no evidence of persistent vaccine-derived poliovirus circulation (World Health Assembly, 1988). Although eradication may eventually be certified, it is likely that poliovirus will never be completely contained, and recent findings indicate that vaccine-derived polioviruses can circulate and cause disease. Consequently, vaccination will probably not be discontinued anytime in the foreseeable future.

Although the use of live, attenuated polio vaccine (OPV) has been crucial to the success of the eradication program thus far, unique properties of the vaccine complicate the decision to cease vaccination. Before we can stop vaccination, we must answer the following questions:

1. How long will OPV persist after it is no longer administered to humans? Will such persistence (including virus excreted by immunocompromised individuals) constitute a threat to the growing number of unvaccinated individuals?
2 What is the transmissibility of OPV strains?
3. Will it be possible to eliminate all potential sources of poliovirus in the post-vaccine era?
4. How will we respond to an outbreak of polio in the post-vaccine era?

Poliovirus infections, which are transmitted by fecal-oral contamination, begin in the pharyngeal and intestinal mucosa before spreading to the blood and invading the central nervous system. Paralytic disease, which occurs in about 1 in 100 infections, results from the destruction of motor neurons. Poliomyelitis can be prevented by the use of either an injected, formalin-inactivated vaccine (inactivated polio vaccine, IPV), or a live, attenuated vaccine which is taken orally and replicates in the intestine (oral polio vaccine, OPV). Both vaccines generate humoral immunity, but only OPV produces local antibodies in the intestine. As a result, wild poliovirus can replicate in the gut of individuals immunized with IPV, but not in the gut of those immunized with OPV.

The OPV strains used in the WHO eradication effort were developed by Albert Sabin, who identified variants of the three poliovirus serotypes that were immunogenic but did not cause disease. Since then, molecular biological tools have been used to identify the mutations responsible for the attenuation phenotypes of the vaccine strains. In the 1980s, scientists discovered that these mutations revert to pathogenicity during replication in the human gut, which explains why OPV-shed virus is more neurovirulent than the administered parent virus.

Will virulent, OPV-derived viruses shed by vaccinees be a threat in the post-vaccination era? To answer this question, we must first consider how long these viruses persist in the environment. In a recent study carried out in Japan, neurovirulent, OPV-derived viruses were isolated from sewage and river water up to three months after routine immunization (Yoshida et al., 2000). The authors concluded that there is an environmental risk of vaccine-associated polio as long as live vaccine is not replaced by inactivated vaccine. Similar studies in Cuba suggest that OPV may persist in the population for several months after vaccination. During the type 3 polio epidemic in Finland in 1984, OPV was detected up to six months after mass immunization. All of these studies were conducted in communities with a high proportion of immune individuals; it is not known if the level of immunity to poliovirus affects the duration of persistence.

The problem of OPV persistence is further complicated by the observation that immunocompromised individuals who receive OPV may excrete virus for extended periods. For example, in one study, a patient who received monotypic Sabin type 3 in 1962 excreted neurovirulent type 3 virus for 637 days with no symptoms of polio (Martin et al., 2000). Individuals with B cell deficiencies often go undiagnosed and may excrete enteroviruses for long periods. The extent to which immunodeficient individuals are infected with polio is unknown and needs to be determined.

After the cessation of polio immunization, OPV will likely continue to circulate in most populations for at least a few months, perhaps up to a year. At the same time, the number of susceptible individuals will increase. This raises the questions: will OPV-derived viruses pose a threat to unvaccinated individuals, and can OPV-derived viruses be transmitted and cause disease in humans?

As long as OPV has been in use, scientists have recognized its transmissibility among humans. Numerous studies have documented the development of anti-poliovirus antibodies in nonimmunized persons in communities undergoing vaccination. For example, in one study of a U.S. Amish community where many individuals refuse vaccination, 89% of unvaccinated children developed antibodies to type 2 poliovirus, presumably from circulation of the vaccine virus from neighboring areas where the vaccine was used. This ability to immunize non-vaccinated individuals is considered to be an advantage of OPV, especially in Third World countries where immunization levels are low and poor sanitation promotes extensive virus spread. However, in the post-eradication era, live vaccine strain transmissibility will be a liability. It will be ironic if it becomes necessary to continue vaccination as protection against vaccine-derived polioviruses.

Several recent studies confirm that OPV-like strains excreted after immunization can be transmitted and cause poliomyelitis among humans. In 2000, a neurovirulent derivative of the Sabin type 2 OPV strain was isolated from sewage in Israel (Shulman et al., 2000). The extent of sequence divergence of this strain from Sabin type 2 indicates that it had probably been replicating in one or more people for at least six years. These observations indicate that OPV-like virus can be transmitted "silently," i.e., in the absence of disease, in an immunized population. In Egypt, 32 polio cases that occurred from 1988–1993 have been attributed to a type 2 vaccine-derived poliovirus strain (Centers for Disease Control and Prevention [CDC], 2001). Analysis of the virus isolate sequences indicates that they were probably derived from a single infection in 1982, the progeny of which circulated in Egypt for the next 10 years. During July and November 2000, an outbreak of poliomyelitis occurred in Hispaniola (CDC, 2000). The virus responsible for this outbreak was derived from the Sabin type 1 strain. Sequence analysis indicates that it had been circulating in the region for approximately two years. All of these findings demonstrate that neurovirulent revertants of OPV can be transmitted among humans and cause poliomyelitis. In light of this information, it is impossible at this time to plan cessation of immunization against polio.

In order to prevent reintroduction of the virus in the post-vaccination era, a crucial component of the eradication effort is the identification and destruction of poliovirus stocks. It will be an enormous task to track down every poliovirus stock, particularly in light of the absence of an enforcement authority. We cannot simply depend on the good will of nations, as suggested by WHO. An even greater challenge is identifying clinical laboratories that unknowingly harbor poliovirus. Finally, how do we deal with a situation in which, for example, a tube labeled "Coxsackievirus B3" actually contains poliovirus type 2? Since this has actually occurred, it is not a hypothetical threat but a real possibility.

A paradox that arises in the post-OPV era is that it will be critically important to continue producing vaccine stocks for use in the event of a disease outbreak. In populations that have lost immunity to the virus, a poliovirus vaccine production facility will be a hazard equivalent to a bioweapons plant. With smallpox, this problem was avoided because of the strain differences between the vaccine and wild viruses, but poliovirus vaccines do not offer such an easy solution.

Which poliovirus vaccine will be produced in the post-OPV era? Because the inactivated polio vaccine (IPV) is produced from wild-type strains of poliovirus, its production would require a high containment facility. Alternatively, IPV might be produced from the Sabin poliovirus strains, although some research would be required to demonstrate the feasibility of this approach. However, immunization with IPV would not prevent intestinal carriage of the virus, increasing the likelihood of spread of the virus in the population. Vaccination with OPV would probably be more effective in curtailing epidemics of poliomyelitis, but excretion of vaccine-derived OPV would be problematic for reasons discussed above.

There are no easy answers to these questions, but it is disturbing that a detailed plan for poliovirus vaccine production in the post-OPV era has not been formulated. Failure to present a coherent plan for the production of vaccine stocks in the post-vaccination world is another reason why we cannot stop vaccinating.

The plan to eradicate polio has had an unfortunate effect on poliovirus research. As noted recently in an article entitled "Don't Underestimate the Enemy" in *Nature*, January 18, 2001, "When an infectious disease appears to be in decline the agent that causes it tends to disappear from the biomedical research agenda." In the late 1990s, WHO and CDC began informing polio research laboratories that they would soon be required to cease poliovirus research and destroy virus and infectious DNA stocks. Although the exact date was somewhat vague, the resulting uncertainty inhibited poliovirus research. Graduate students and postdoctoral fellows no longer viewed working on poliovirus as a wise career option, and funding agencies and their peer review groups began to question the wisdom of long-term (five-year) investment in research programs on the virus. This effect was unfortunate, because many projects relevant to the eradication effort—work on new vaccines, animal models for virus transmission, and anti-viral compounds (which might be useful in a post-vaccination-era outbreak of polio)—did not proceed. WHO decided not to continue poliovirus research in 1988 because the virus would be eradicated by 2000!

Today it is quite clear to many virologists that it might not be possible to eliminate poliovirus from the world. It therefore seems unfortunate that the poliovirus research establishment has been substantially depleted, especially since questions relevant to the eradication effort have not been adequately addressed. One of the lessons we have learned from the polio eradication effort is that there continues to be a large gap between basic research and public health. For example, the research community has doubted whether it will be possible to eliminate poliovirus ever since the eradication goal was first announced in 1988. Nevertheless, the force of public health policy has overriden these concerns, resulting in the dismantling of research programs that could otherwise have contributed to the eradication effort. Future eradication campaigns should benefit from this experience. Although it is important to convince governments and health authorities that a disease can be eradicated, it is also important to maintain communication with the research community so that crucial research continues.

ANTIVIRAL THERAPY IN THE MANAGEMENT OF POST-ERADICATION INFECTIOUS DISEASE OUTBREAKS

Richard J. Whitley, M.D.

Loeb Eminent Scholar Chair and Professor, Department of Pediatrics
University of Alabama at Birmingham, Birmingham, AL

Prevention must take precedence over treatment of infectious diseases. In an age of unparalleled successful vaccination, particularly when the eradication of smallpox has been documented and the eradication of poliovirus is anticipated, one must question the necessity of developing antiviral drugs targeting infectious diseases slated for global eradication. Successful immunization against measles, mumps, rubella, diphtheria, and many other pathogens has been demonstrated worldwide, though with varying degrees of success.

There are several different circumstances under which re-emergence of an infectious agent might be anticipated:

- Bioterrorism (e.g., deployment of smallpox),
- Resurgence of an infection thought to be eradicated (e.g., poliomyelitis in Santo Domingo), and
- Clinical reactivation of a vaccine-preventable latent virus (e.g., varicella) transmitted to a high-risk susceptible (seronegative) individual.

This overview focuses on the potential utility of specific antiviral and more generalized broad-spectrum antiviral agents in a post-eradication vaccine era.

Available Therapeutic Resources

The armamentarium of the public health physician with regard to antiviral agents is limited, at best. Successful antiviral therapy has only been demonstrated in four general infectious areas:

1. The management of influenza virus infections with tricyclic amines and neuraminidase inhibitors,
2. The treatment of HIV infection with reverse transcriptase inhibitors, protease inhibitors, and other novel therapeutics,
3. The therapy of several herpes virus infections, including herpes simplex virus, cytomegalovirus, and varicella zoster virus, with nucleoside and nucleotide analogs, and
4. Therapeutic interventions for hepatitis B and hepatitis C with nucleoside analogs and interferons.

While therapy for each of these broad infectious disease agents has been shown to be clinically efficacious, resulting in decreased morbidity and mortality, no therapeutic intervention should supplant disease prevention by vaccination. Toward this end, some therapeutic agents have been developed for pre-emptive antiviral therapy to be administered before overt disease but in the presence of viral antigenemia. This approach has proven very successful in the management of cytomegalovirus disease in organ transplant recipients.

Currently, none of the immunological interventions or modulators (e.g., interferon or interferon-like compounds) have proven valuable in the prevention of viral disease. With the exception of limited monoclonal antibodies (e.g., palivizumab for respiratory syncytial viruses), disease prevention has not been achieved by this modality.

Public Health Implications

With the exception of influenza and HIV infections, those diseases for which antiviral therapy exists are not usually considered epidemic. Diseases that could take on epidemic proportions—namely, smallpox, measles, rubella, polio, dengue, and Ebola—have never been considered candidates for antiviral drug development. This is alarming in light of the fact that extremist governments or individuals will likely consider using these agents as bioterrorist weapons in the post-vaccine eradication era when seroprotection will have waned in the community at large.

Scientists have identified molecular targets amenable to the development of selective and specific antiviral agents. The knowledge of viral-host interactions should lead to the development of specific and more generalized modulators of host response, such as induction of intracellular interferon pathways.

The unique properties of each virus need to be considered when developing selective, specific inhibitors to viral replication. For example, several viruses—primarily the herpes viruses but also hepatitis B and C—have a propensity to establish latency. Recognizing that reactivation can occur, even with an effective vaccine, exposure of susceptible (seronegative) or non-vaccinated individuals could result in exaggerated disease. An example of this is the reactivation of varicella zoster virus which results in shingles, or chickenpox. Shingles is contagious for seronegative individuals and is always more severe in adults than in children.

Changes in the antigenic nature of an organism may also render it more pathogenic for the population at large. This phenomenon has already been documented by the detection of the H5N1 influenza A strain in Hong Kong. It is anticipated that a major antigenic shift in the near future will result in a worldwide influenza pandemic. The lack of adequate vaccine stores and vaccines containing the appropriate antigens, combined with the inability to generate sufficient quantities of antiviral drugs, would leave the world's population at significant risk for disease caused by pandemic influenza.

Conclusion

In an era of rapid vaccine deployment and committed attempts at worldwide eradication of diseases other than smallpox, questions regarding the need to develop additional antiviral agents are very serious. With the lingering threat of bioterrorism, the availability of therapeutics to treat vaccine-preventable diseases, such as smallpox, should be considered a high priority.

It is impossible to envision a universal vaccine program for the prevention of such diseases as rabies, Ebola, dengue, and others. However, all of these viruses are amenable to the development of specific antiviral agents.

Molecular biology tools are now available for the development of antiviral agents. Plus, the knowledge derived from developing therapeutics for one virus can be applied to other viruses. For example, therapeutics directed against polio can be applied to other members of the Picornavirus family, including hepatitis A virus, rhinoviruses, enteroviruses, and coxsackieviruses, all of which cause significant morbidity in the world's population. Toward this end, the pharmaceutical industry must make a commitment to the development of antiviral interventions.

POTENTIAL USE OF CYTOKINES AND ANTIBODY FOR POST-EXPOSURE PROPHYLAXIS IN THE POST-ERADICATION ERA

Diane E. Griffin, M.D., Ph.D.

Professor and Chair, W. Harry Feinstone Department of Molecular Microbiology and Immunology

Johns Hopkins School of Hygiene and Public Health, Baltimore, MD

An important benefit of viral eradication, in addition to elimination of morbidity and mortality due to infection, is the elimination of the need for continued immunization of large numbers of people. Discontinuation of universal immunization will result in considerable cost savings. However, it will also eventually create a population susceptible to widespread infection in the event of reintroduction or re-emergence of the eradicated virus. Because reintroduction will always be a possibility, even in the best-controlled circumstances, it is necessary to have a planned response if and when it should occur. There are several possible responses:

- Resumption of widespread immunization, assuming that the vaccine and vaccine-manufacturing capacity are available.
- The use of antiviral drugs for prophylaxis or treatment (see previous section of this chapter).
- The use of immunoprophylaxis for protection, including both nonspecific approaches to stimulation of innate antiviral defenses and specific prophylaxis directed at particular pathogens.

Nonspecific Inhibition of Virus Replication

The first line of defense against viral infection is the innate immune response. Innate defenses not only act to control virus replication early after infection, but they also shape and influence the nature of subsequent specific immune responses. This continuum between the innate and acquired immune responses to pathogens is increasingly being recognized. Many important components of the innate immune response contribute to the early control of viral replication. The best understood is interferon (IFN), a cytokine which is produced by many types of cells and was first recognized for its ability to make previously susceptible cells resistant to infection by a wide variety of viruses. In addition to the first recognized IFN, now known as type I or IFN α/β, there are several other cytokines with important antiviral properties. Cytokines produced early after infection include type II IFN or IFN-γ, which is produced by natural killer (NK) cells, and tumor necrosis factor (TNF)γ, which is produced by phagocytic cells such as macrophages.

Current knowledge and therapeutic experience is most extensive for type I IFN, which induces an antiviral cellular state by interacting with the IFN α/β receptor, IFNAR. IFNAR signals through a pathway involving transcription factors STAT-1 and STAT-2 to induce transcription of a large number of IFN-responsive genes and subsequent production of antiviral proteins. The best studied of these proteins and pathways are those involving the dsRNA-activated protein kinase, PKR, which inhibits protein synthesis; the dsRNA-activated oligoadenylate system, which degrades RNA; and the MX GTPases, which inhibit RNA synthesis. In addition to these direct antiviral responses, IFN also upregulates expression of major histocompatibility complex (MHC) molecules on the cell surface, thereby enhancing recognition from cells involved in inducing an immunologically specific immune response. From extensive study of these IFN-regulated pathways, several facts are clear:

1. The pathways described to date involve only a small proportion of the messages known to be induced by IFN (i.e., IFN α/β probably induces about 90 different pathways).

2. Each pathway affects replication to a different degree, depending on the particular virus. A pathway that interferes with the replication of one virus may have absolutely no effect on the replication of another virus.

3. Our understanding of how IFN inhibits viral replication is incomplete.

4. Viruses have evolved a large number of mechanisms to counteract the effects of IFN. These mechanisms may or may not be preserved in the tissue culture-adapted virus strains most often used for study.

Several recombinant forms of both IFN-α and IFN-β are currently available and licensed for treatment of a variety of diseases, including multiple sclerosis, lymphoid tumors, and chronic viral infections (particularly hepatitis B and hepatitis C). Therefore, we have knowledge of dosing and side effects for prophylaxis against chronic infections in humans. However, our experience with prophylaxis against acute infections is very limited. IFN has been used locally for prophylaxis against upper respiratory infections, and, although effective, often causes side effects resembling symptoms of the disease being prevented. Many people would rather have a cold than suffer these side effects. Experience with preventing systemic infections is limited to animal models, where efficacy can be demonstrated as long as the IFN or IFN-inducer (e.g., poly IC) is administered before or shortly after exposure to the virus. Therefore, although our experience with this approach is limited, prophylactic use of IFN is certainly a rational approach to protection from infection early after exposure. However, its effectiveness against the specific wild-type virus of interest would need to be confirmed.

As mentioned above, viruses have evolved many ways to circumvent host cell antiviral activities (Alcami and Koszinowski, 2000). For example, viruses from many different families (e.g., picornaviruses, rhabdoviruses, reoviruses, retroviruses, orthomyxoviruses, adenoviruses, herpesviruses, poxviruses) block the activation of the PKR pathway by either producing decoy RNAs, binding dsRNA, or degrading PKR protein. These mechanisms are especially prevalent in wild-type viruses, whose ability to escape the effects of IFN is likely to be important for virulence and transmission. As another example, the virulent myxomatosis in the poxvirus family produces proteins that bind host TNF, IFN, and a broad range of chemokines. Because viral defenses against host innate immune responses are not necessary for viral replication *in vitro*, they may be lost, not expressed, or mutated in tissue culture-adapted strains of virus. However, they are very important for *in vivo* virulence.

In addition to IFN α/β, other less well-studied antiviral cytokines include IFN-γ and TNFα. *In vitro,* both exhibit antiviral activity against some viruses in some cells, but their effects are much more variable that those of

IFN a/b. "Upstream" inducers of these effector cytokines, such as IL-12 or immunostimulatory oligonucleotides, could potentially be developed as broadly active prophylactic agents. However, considerable research on toxicity and effectiveness would need to be performed before any of these agents could be considered for widespread prophylactic use.

Specific Inhibition of Virus Replication

Acquired immune responses provide specific protection against re-infection by many viral pathogens and, as such, serve as the basis for protection by immunization. In the pre-immunization era, immune globulin containing polyclonal antibodies to specific viruses was used for prevention and treatment for a number of infections (Ordman et al., 1944). For both polio and measles, data from excellent controlled studies show that passive prophylaxis can prevent disease in outbreak situations; protection can last for weeks after a single dose. Some of these data have been used to determine what levels of antiviral antibody need to be induced by vaccines in order to provide protection from infection.

However, there are a couple of serious problems with passive transfer of immune globulin. First, the amount of antibody against the virus may be relatively low but the volume needed relatively large. This problem will be exacerbated as the population's immunity to the virus wanes following eradication and cessation of immunization. Second, using large pools of donors to generate the immune globulin carries the risk of transmitting other infectious agents.

Fortunately, there has been considerable progress on this front since the early days when immune globulin was used for passive protection against polio and measles. This is illustrated by the current products available for prophylaxis against respiratory syncytial virus (RSV), a cause of serious lower respiratory disease in young infants, particularly those with cardiac and pulmonary abnormalities.

There is no vaccine for RSV. Passive transfer of immune globulin is protective, but not all infants can tolerate the volume loads required to achieve protective antibody levels (PREVENT, 1997). More effective and potent prophylactic products have been developed and licensed. In particular, animal studies have shown that a mouse monoclonal antibody (MAb) provides protection against RSV by binding to the F protein. Determinants of antibody specificity lie in the variable complementary determining regions (CDRs) of MAb's Fab H and L chains. But the rest of the mouse MAb molecule induces an immune response in humans. Through genetic engineering, mouse MAb has been "humanized" so that every region of the molecule, except for those portions of the CDRs that determine specificity for binding to the RSV F protein, are now human. Humanized MAb provides effective prophylaxis against severe RSV-induced disease (The Impact-RSV Study Group, 1998).

With recent technological improvements, variable regions of human antibodies with desired specificity can be cloned directly from antibody-secreting cells in the blood or bone marrow (Hoogenboom and Chames, 2000; Little et al., 2000). These clones can then be cloned into another vector and converted directly into whole human IgG molecules (Sanna et al., 1999). By knowing which antibody specificities are protective against eradicated viruses, clinically useful immunoprophylactic reagents could be generated relatively easily. These antibodies would then be available for production and use in the event of reintroduction or re-emergence of an eradicated virus.

Conclusion

Immunomodulators that would be broadly protective against viral infections—such as IFN α/β, TNFα, and immunostimulatory DNA—are in the early stages of development. IFN α/β is the best characterized but has been used primarily for treatment of chronic viral infections, not prophylaxis against acute viral infections. Humanized MAbs have proven successful at preventing acute viral infections and are currently being used as a prophylaxis against RSV. Technology has advanced to a point where specific prophylactic MAbs could be developed for use against other viral pathogens besides RSV, but this has not been done for polio, measles, or smallpox.

Given the diversity of viruses, it seems unlikely that a universal prophylactic agent will be identified. Rather, studies will need to focus on developing prophylaxis for those infections deemed to pose the greatest risks. Prophylactic agents must be developed before they are needed in the post-eradication era.

THE POTENTIAL ROLE OF PROBIOTICS AND MICROBIAL ECOLOGY IN HOST DEFENSE

Susanna Cunningham-Rundles, Ph.D.

Professor of Immunology, Department of Pediatrics
Weill Medical College of Cornell University, New York, NY

The human immune system provides host defense against sudden invasion from exogenous pathogenic microorganisms and viruses, while simultaneously maintaining continual surveillance against incursion from endogenous microbes. Immunization will create a specific pathogen-free environment only if there is a continuous normal immune response within an immunized majority of the community. An apparently healthy person's response to vaccine is often taken for granted, even though detailed knowledge of the normal immune response is lacking. There has been little consideration given to the possibility that the human immune system may be affected by selective pressure from changing world conditions. As immunity wanes, even immunized individuals may be highly vulnerable in the absence of total eradication. Immunity in the community at large is not determined by the poor response to some vaccines by young children and immunocompromised persons if the proportionate representation of these groups is small. However, the increasing size of this poor response population—for example in parts of the world with a high incidence of HIV infection—may significantly affect whether standard immunization practices can lead to the eradication of infectious pathogens.

The strength of the immune system is both challenged and maintained through continual interaction with an internal microbial milieu. Understanding this fundamental interaction will provide new insights into what makes an immune response functional and will likely lead to novel approaches to restoring or enhancing immune function.

In healthy people, microflora are normally present on all external surfaces and the internal surfaces of the upper respiratory tract, gastrointestinal tract, perineum, vagina and distal urethra. They are usually absent from the internal surfaces of the bronchi, alveolar spaces, urinary tract, and uterus, as well as the blood, deep tissues, organs, and brain.

Within the gut, there are distinct, closely regulated differences in the relative density of bacteria. Mechanisms that mediate and maintain these regional differences include physical structures, such as the glottis; physiological barriers, such as gastric pH; and the continual action of both the innate and adaptive immune systems. The normal human gut is persistently colonized. Since there is no fixed boundary between colonization and infection, response to persistent colonization likely involves repeated waves of immune activation. Thus, gastrointestinal colonization conditions the activation potential of the immune system.

The gut immune system operates independently of the systemic immune system, and the gut's resident T cells have developed specialized functional capacities independent of thymic influence. Recent studies (Gill et al., 2000; Macpherson et al., 2000; Walker, 2000) have shown that the gastrointestinal–immune interface is a frontier zone, and the gut's local innate response to antigenic or pathogenic challenge has a surprisingly strong influence on the systemic immune response. A key mediator for this response is the natural killer, or NK, cell. NK cells are characterized by their spontaneous ability to kill tumor or virally infected cells. They also produce cytokines, which regulate host defense against bacteria and influence the development of the adaptive immune system. NK cells begin functioning at birth, when microbial colonization of the gut occurs. In the early post-birth period, neonatal NK cells show absent or decreased cytolytic activity against the reference erythroleukemia tumor cell target K562. However, as demonstrated in Figure 5-1, certain bacteria can directly activate the neonatal NK cell system. This functional response is accompanied by *de novo* induction of gamma interferon production. The preparations of bacteria used in these studies—ImuVert (ribosomal vesicles from *Serratia marscesens*) and OK432 (whole inactivated *Streptococcus pyogenes*)—have broad immunoadjuvant properties. These experiments *in vitro* mirror what happens *in vivo* in response to conventional environmental microbes. This

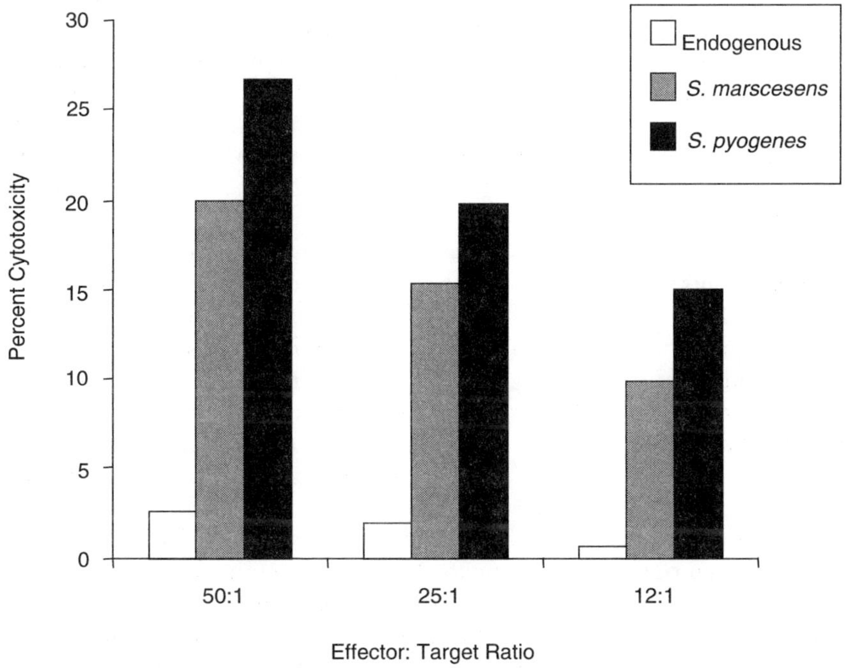

FIGURE 5-1 Stimulation of neonatal natural killer cell activity by bacteria. This shows the effect of *S. marscesens* and *S. pyogenes* on NK activity of peripheral blood mononuclear cells in the short-term Cr^{51} release assay against K562. Data are given as percent specific release at three effector target ratios. (Cunningham-Rundles and Nesin in "Persistent Bacterial Infections," 2000, reprinted with permission from ASM Press)

unique response to bacteria probably evolved to provide a transition between the pre-natal suppression of fetal immune effector activity, which is necessary for the maintenance of maternal fetal tolerance, and the post-natal requirement for rapid response toward potential microbial pathogens.

Microflora directly alter the architecture and physiology of the mucosa by inducing an immune response, which they probably continue to influence and regulate throughout life. Emerging studies (Wold and Adlerberth, 2000) have suggested that the specific composition of microflora is highly varied among different cultures and that it tends to remain constant for the individual once established after birth. Normal flora do not directly harm the normal host; plus they contain commensals which produce nutrients, absorbable peptides, and vitamins, all of which benefit the host. It is now possible to study the potential significance of this lifelong interaction, thanks to the advent of genetic typing, which spurred investigation of flora comprised of species resistant to current culturing methods. One study (Ahrne et al., 1998) showed that the well-characterized beneficent commensals, such as lactobacilli, form a small and rather fragile part of the overall flora. The ecology of microflora is strongly influenced by oxygen tolerance. Commensal bacteria are primarily obligate anaerobes, whereas key pathogenic bacteria are facultative anaerobes that replicate faster in the presence of oxygen. Thus lactobacilli and bifididobacteria, which are normal gut commensals, survive and replicate in the presence of oxygen but not as effectively as, for example, *E. coli*.

If beneficial microbes have a selective advantage, their colonization may prevent outgrowth of more pathogenic bacteria. Although Metchnikoff proposed in 1907 (Metchnikoff, 1907) that lactic acid bacteria would have a favorable effect on health, the concept of probiotic bacteria—living microbes introduced into the body to improve intestinal microbial balance—is recent (Fuller, 1989). Probiotic bacteria have proven effective against antibiotic-associated diarrhea and certain persistent and clinically significant infections, such as *C. difficile*. Experimental studies (Bergogne-Berezin, 2000; Hirayama and Rafter, 1999; Hove et al., 1999; Kirjavainen et al., 1999; Majamaa et al., 1995) have shown that probiotic lactobacilli can neutralize carcinogens, replace microflora that produce carcinogens and tumor promoters, and produce antitumor factors through direct actions in the gastrointestinal tract. Essential characteristics for efficacy include resistance to acid and bile and ability to colonize and adhere to the colonic mucosa (Bengmark, 1999). Moreover, current studies (Cunningham-Rundles et al., 2000; Devi et al., 1999; Hessle et al., 1999) have suggested that probiotic lactobacilli may serve as immunoadjuvants, thereby increasing weak systemic immune response, even in the HIV+ host. Possible mechanisms of action include competition for specific ecological niches, immunological stimulation of the mucosal barrier, and induction of specific cytokine patterns.

Thus, probiotic bacteria have strong potential to sustain natural immune response towards environmental pathogens in the post-vaccine era. Additionally, probiotic lactobacillus may prove useful in strengthening immune responses in persons whose host defense capacity has been compromised by chronic infection or short-term stressors. However, there are a few key questions concerning the use of probiotic bacteria in the immunodeficient host, including:

- Can the immune-deficient host develop a normal immune response towards lactobacillus?
- Is this response qualitatively or quantitatively different from that of immunocompetent persons?
- Are there safety issues, such as potential for translocation?

The most extreme example of acquired immune deficiency is HIV infection. Normal bacterial flora are altered in HIV infection, as evident by the frequency of bacteremia associated with altered gastrointestinal function, diarrhea, and malabsorption. Failure-to-thrive is relatively common in congenital HIV infection and is linked to altered gastrointestinal function and chronic cytokine activation. Our lab studies the effect of *L. plantarum 299v,* a specially developed probiotic lactobacillus, on growth and specific systemic immune response following oral supplementation in the HIV+ child. There appears to be a generally beneficial effect on immune response. Surprisingly, the HIV+ children's level of cross-reacting immune response to *LP299*, as a group prior to supplementation, is essentially independent of CD4+ T cell percentage, which is unlike response to any other activator. Data are shown in Figure 5-2. Children who did not respond to *LP299v* before supplementation did develop response after supplementation; the oral supplement was well tolerated, colonization was temporary, and there were no side effects. The mechanism of action is currently under study; preliminary data suggest that treatment promotes a T helper type 1 cytokine response.

These studies support current interest in commensal bacteria as antigen-delivery vehicles, as well as potential adjuvants. The possibility that modulation of gastrointestinal flora might be used to strengthen immune response is especially relevant for protection of future populations against emerging infections in a post-immunization era where, paradoxically, the immune system may face even greater challenges.

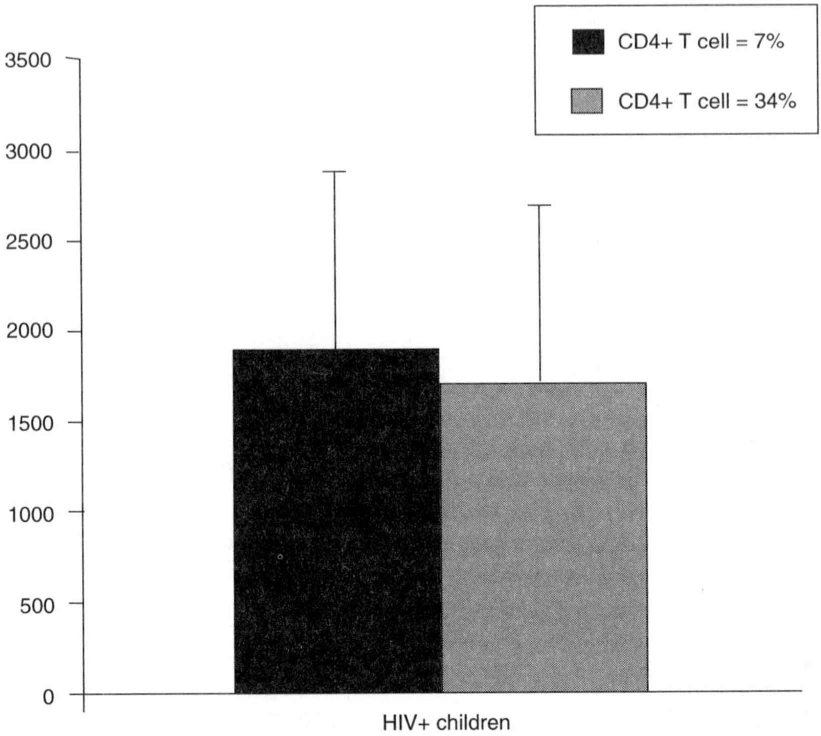

FIGURE 5-2 Immune response to *Lactobacillus plantarum 299v* in HIV+ children in relationship to CD4+ T cells. Peripheral blood mononuclear cells were cultured in a microtiter plate assay and pulse labeled with ^{3}H thymidine. Data show mean net maximum response to *LP299v* antigen in children grouped by CD4+ T cell level. (Cunningham-Rundles and Nesin in "Persistent Bacterial Infections," 2000, reprinted with permission from ASM Press.)

REFERENCES

Ahrne S, Nobaek S, Jeppsson B, Adlerberth I, Wold AE, and Molin G. 1998. The normal Lactobacillus flora of healthy human oral and rectal mucosa. *Journal of Applied Microbiology* 85:88–94.

Alcami A and Koszinowski UH. 2000. Viral mechanisms of immune evasion. *Trends in Microbiology* 8:410–418.

Bengmark S. 1999. Gut microenvironment and immune function. *Current Opinion in Clinical Nutrition and Metabolic Care* 2:83–85.

Bergogne-Berezin E. 2000. Treatment and prevention of antibiotic associated diarrhea. *International Journal of Antimicrobial Agents* 16(4):521–526.

Centers for Disease Control and Prevention. 2000. Outbreak of poliomyelitis—Dominican Republic and Haiti, 2000. *Morbidity and Mortality Weekly Report* 49:1094, 1103.

Centers for Disease Control and Prevention. 2001. Circulation of a type 2 vaccine-derived poliovirus—Egypt, 1982–1993. *Morbidity and Mortality Weekly Report* 50(3):41–2, 51.

Cunningham-Rundles S, Ahrne S, Bengmark S, Johann-Liang R, Marshall F, Metakis L, Califano C, Dunn AM, Grassey C, Hinds G, and Cervia J. 2000. Probiotics and immune response. *American Journal of Gastroenterology* 95(1 Suppl):S22–S25.

Devi S, Yasoda Devi P, and Prakash MS. 1999. Effect of Lactobacillus supplementation on immune status of malnourished pre-school children. *Indian Journal of Pediatrics* 66(5):663–668.

Fuller, R. 1989. Probiotics in man and animals. *Journal of Applied Bacteriology* 66:365–378.

Gill HS, Rutherfurd KJ, Prasad J, and Gopal PK. 2000. Enhancement of natural and acquired immunity by Lactobacillus rhamnosus (HN001), Lactobacillus acidophilus (HN017) and Bifidobacterium lactis (HN019). *British Journal of Nutrition* 83:167–176.

Hessle C, Hanson LA, and Wold AE. 1999. Lactobacilli from human gastrointestinal mucosa are strong stimulators of IL-12 production. *Clinical and Experimental Immunology* 116(2):276–282.

Hirayama K and Rafter J. 1999. The role of lactic acid bacteria in colon cancer prevention: Mechanistic considerations. *Antonie van Leeuwenhoek* 76:391–394.

Hoogenboom HR and Chames P. 2000. Natural and designer binding sites made by phage display technology. *Immunology Today* 21:371–378.

Hove H, Norgaard H, and Mortensen PB. 1999. Lactic acid bacteria and the human gastrointestinal tract. *European Journal of Clinical Nutrition* 53:339–350.

The Impact-RSV Study Group. 1998. Palivizumab, a humanized respiratory syncytial virus monoclonal antibody, reduces hospitalization from respiratory syncytial virus infection in high-risk infants. *Pediatrics* 102:531–537.

Kirjavainen PV, Apostolou E, Salminen SJ, and Isolauri E. 1999. New aspects of probiotics—A novel approach in the management of food allergy. *Allergy* 54(9):909–915.

Little M, Kipriyanov SM, LeGall F, and Moldenhauer G. 2000. Of mice and men: Hybridoma and recombinant antibodies. *Immunology Today* 21:364–370.

Macpherson AJ, Gatto D, Sainsbury E, Harriman GR, Hengartner H, and Zinkernagel RM. 2000. A primitive T cell-independent mechanism of intestinal mucosal IgA responses to commensal bacteria. *Science* 288:2222–2226.

Majamaa H, Isolauri E, Saxelin M, and Vesikari T. 1995. Lactic acid bacteria in the treatment of acute rotavirus gastroenteritis. *Journal of Pediatric Gastroenterology and Nutrition* 20(3):333–338.

Martin J, Dunn G, Hull R, Patel V, and Minor PD. 2000. Evolution of the Sabin strain of type 3 poliovirus in an immunodeficient patient during the entire 637-day period of virus excretion. *Journal of Virology* 74(7):3001–3010.

Metchnikoff E. 1907. *The Prolongation of Life*. London: Heinemann.

Nataro JP, Blazer MJ, Cunningham-Rundles S, eds. 2000. *Persistent Bacterial Infections*. Washington, DC: American Society of Microbiology Press. 500 pp.

Ordman CW, Jennings CG, and Janeway CA. 1944. Chemical, clinical and immunological studies on the products of human plasma fractionation. XII. The use of concentrated normal human serum gamma globulin (human immune serum globulin) in the prevention and attenuation of measles. *Journal of Clinical Investigation* 23:541–549.

The PREVENT Study Group. 1997. Reduction of respiratory syncytial virus hospitalization among premature infants and infants with bronchopulmonary dysplasia using respiratory syncytial virus immune globulin prophylaxis. *Pediatrics* 99:93–99.

Sanna PP, Samson ME, Moon JS, Rozenshteyn R, De Logu A, Williamson RA, and Burton DR. 1999. pFab-CMV, a single vector system for the rapid conversion of recombinant Fabs into whole IgG1 antibodies. *Immunotechnology* 4:185–188.

Shulman LM, Manor Y, Handsher R, Delpeyroux F, McDonough MJ, Halmut T, Silberstein I, Alfandari J, Quay J, Fisher T, Robinov J, Kew OM, Crainic R, and Mendelson E. 2000. Molecular and antigenic characterization of a highly evolved derivative of the type 2 oral poliovaccine strain isolated from sewage in Israel. *Journal of Clinical Microbiology* 38(10):3729–3734.

Walker WA. 2000. Role of nutrients and bacterial colonization in the development of intestinal host defense. *Journal of Pediatric Gastroenterology and Nutrition* 30:S2–S7.

Wold A and Adlerberth I. 2000. Pathological consequences of commensalism. In Nataro JP, Blaser MJ, and Cunningham-Rundles S, (eds.). *Persistent Bacterial Infections*, pp. 145–163. Washington, DC: American Society of Microbiology Press.

World Health Assembly. 1988. *Global Eradication of Poliomyelitis by the Year 2000.* Geneva: World Health Organization.

Yoshida H, Horie H, Matsuura K, and Miyamura T. 2000. Characterisation of vaccine-derived polioviruses isolated from sewage and river water in Japan. *Lancet* 356(9240):1461–1463.

6

The Challenges to Post-Eradication Outbreaks

OVERVIEW

As the United States enters the post-eradication era, it is critical that we develop thoughtful institutional strategies to meet the challenges of potential reintroduction or re-emergence of disease. The waning of surveillance and laboratory diagnostic capability, reduced medical awareness, lack of vaccine supply and production capacity, limited institutional response capacity, decreased immunity in the population at large, and increased threats of bioterrorism all leave the non-immunized populace highly vulnerable to a post-eradication outbreak. Planning for the post-eradication era will likely warrant consideration of major outbreak scenarios and the required capacity for response.

Hospitals serve as a major hub in the U.S. health care system and can and should play a major role in an outbreak response. However, they have neither the capacity nor infrastructure to handle such a crisis, and there are no financial incentives or mandates in place to encourage them to devote efforts to anticipate potential outbreak scenarios. There is an enormous amount of work to be done to prepare hospitals for the post-eradication era.

Because of the increasing threat of bioterrorism, especially with regard to smallpox, planning for potential outbreaks in a post-eradication era should involve consideration of national security implications in addition to public health considerations. Although health care workers would be the sentinels of any outbreak response, no matter what the security implications, a bioterrorist act may require the involvement of other communities, such as intelligence and defense and arms control, that may not typically be involved in outbreak response. The appropriate agencies and institutions must be prepared to offer a swift and effective collaborative response.

Preparing for unexpected disease outbreaks also requires a flexible and adaptive post-eradication vaccine program involving continued vaccine production, research, and development. Vaccine manufacture must keep up with changing regulatory requirements (e.g., safety issues concerning the threat of prion-mediated diseases from animal protein components of vaccines), new scientific challenges (e.g., alterations to the virus), and changes in the manufacturing process.

Institutions must be prepared to deal with the psychological challenges expected to surface during a post-eradication outbreak, namely, fear and panic. Well-trained responder staff, effective communication regarding the risks of infection and exposure, and a swift, well-coordinated public health response will be key in promoting a healthy public reaction.

Although U.S. institutions may be starting to take some steps in preparation for a post-eradication era, much of the developing world lags far behind. Many countries are not only still struggling with early eradication initiatives—for example, immunizing all children and developing effective communications networks—they are doing so in the face of adversity. Many developing countries lack not only immunization services but basic health care services as well, and are in the midst of conflict situations where vaccinators are being killed in the field.

This issue of equity has increasingly become a component of global health concerns. Access to limited quantities of vaccines has been debated as a human rights issue. Within the United States, this focus has been on the uninsured and underserved populations. More broadly, in developing countries—where the ability to pay for vaccines and maintain appropriate infrastructure for vaccine delivery remains quite limited—the responsibilities of international organizations, national governments, development banks, and private-sector suppliers are raised as a challenging ethical question.

READY OR NOT: THE U.S. HEALTH CARE SYSTEM AND EMERGING INFECTIONS

Kenneth D. Bloem, M.P.H.

Senior Fellow, The Johns Hopkins University Center for Biodefense Studies, Baltimore, MD, and Former CEO, Georgetown University Medical Center, Washington, DC

The preparedness of the U.S. health care system to respond to future disease outbreaks—accidental or intentional—deserves careful consideration. A caveat may be in order here, however, as this topic will force us to descend from the Olympian heights of scientific discourse to the arid plains of bureaucracies, institutions, and politics. This presentation will focus on hospitals, clinics, and home care agencies—what is commonly termed the "U.S. health care system"—as opposed to the public health system, whose readiness is addressed elsewhere in this report.

To the question, "Are we prepared?" the answer, in my opinion, is emphatically negative. This lack of readiness is characterized by:

- lack of capacity and infrastructure,
- lack of incentives and mandates,
- absence of networks of collaborating institutions, and
- unresolved staffing and legal policy issues.

It is worth noting that there may be legitimate conflicting perspectives on what role the U.S. health care delivery system should play in response to an epidemic that constitutes a major public health threat. This paper supports the notion that the acute health care system can and ought to play a very important, but delimited, role in helping the nation respond to future outbreaks. Following is an assessment of the four problems listed above. Their solutions are critical to an effective health care system response.

Capacity and Infrastructure Issues

In order for the health care system to respond effectively to a potential disease outbreak, the health system must be operating reasonably effectively *prior to* the outbreak. That is, a certain amount of basic functionality, organizational infrastructure strength, and extra capacity (i.e., availability of drugs, equipment, supplies, and personnel) will be a *sine qua non* of an effective response. If hospitals and physicians are already struggling to handle day-to-day operations due to a lack of staff, equipment, and other core capacities, it will be impossible for them to respond effectively to a significant crisis.

Unfortunately, U.S. hospitals are currently experiencing tremendous economic pressures. One-third of all hospitals are losing money. Of the two-thirds that are still profitable, their margins declined by a third between 1998 and 1999. Their profitability is only 4.7%, which is only slightly above the medical Consumer Price Index (CPI). In addition to the Balanced Budget Act of 1997, which reduced aggregate hospitals' Medicare payments by more than Congress intended, hospitals face a host of new regulatory demands including HIPAA (Health Insurance Portability Act), which industry analysts estimate will cost the sector more than did Y2K preparedness efforts. Other regulatory pressures include ergonomic regulations, patient safety regulations, and major seismic upgrades (for California hospitals), to cite just a few.

The problems hospitals currently face are not only financial. The most acute operational issues relate to staff shortages—including nurses, technologists, pharmacists, technicians, nurses' aides, housekeepers, medical records coders, and others. Current staff levels are insufficient for hospitals to cope even with the small and entirely predictable seasonal influenza epidemics. To cite a few examples:

- In December 1999, during the flu season, three-quarters of the Los Angeles emergency rooms were so full that, for 10 days, they had to reroute ambulances to other hospitals.
- In Maryland, the amount of time that hospitals are on "emergency by-pass" has doubled each year for the past three years.
- In San Antonio, the city's Emergency Medical Services physician-director was quoted in a *New York Times* article by C. Goldberg, "Emergency Crews Wary as Hospitals Say, 'No Vacancy,' " December 17, 2000, as saying "We're dying; I got called nine times yesterday to divert my ambulances—and that wasn't an unusual day. We've got an epidemic of the nonavailability of acute care beds, and the epidemic is becoming a pandemic."

Because the population is aging and academic enrollments in key health care professions have declined, most observers are worried that these infrastructure problems will only become worse. In the same *New York Times* article mentioned above, the director of a suburban Boston ER, for example, likened ERs to canaries in the coal mine: "We are basically the canary that's telling the story that the whole system is in trouble, its capacity is inadequate to meet the peak demands."

In addition to chronic infrastructure deficiencies, hospitals lack the capacity to handle "surges" of new patients. For example, a 1998 survey of medical resources for the state of Minnesota revealed that only 60 of 144 acute care hospitals—only 465 beds state-wide—had negative air pressure rooms, which are critical tools for managing patients with highly contagious diseases (Osterholm and Schwartz, 2000). As another example, a recent fire in a downtown high-rise motivated the Maryland Secretary of Health to commission a study which revealed that the city of Baltimore, home to two major medical centers and medical schools, could not handle a situation involving only 100 casualties needing overnight ventilators (O'Toole, 2000).

After two decades of hospital reimbursement policies based exclusively on market principles, hospitals now operate on a "just in time—just what's required" basis which governs the availability of drugs, supplies, equipment, and staffing. In the process, we have lost sight of the historic concept of the hospital as a community resource that is always ready in the event of disease outbreak.

Incentives and Mandates

Among the range of issues with which hospital executives deal on a daily basis, a potential disease outbreak—whether accidental or as a result of bioterrorism—is a low-probability event that competes for attention with more pressing, and more certain, matters. Currently, hospitals have neither incentives, such as funding, to prepare for future outbreaks, nor a legal mandate to do so.

Since the Reagan administration, the United States' policies governing hospital reimbursement have been fundamentally free-market-based. This has led to economic competition among hospitals within a community, as well as the notion that hospitals that support "issues of the commons" (e.g., care for the poor, medical education, biomedical research) without receiving full reimbursement are doing something "economically irrational." Spending significant dollars preparing for bioterrorism, or a similar event on behalf of the community, would trigger a red flag to a hospital's managed care payers, who would think they were overpaying (Bentley, 2000).

This does not imply that hospitals would not respond in the event of a crisis. In fact, American hospitals have a record of extraordinary response when disaster strikes. The point is that, without preparedness funding, it is economically irrational to expect or hope for preparatory efforts on the part of any individual health care organization.

In addition to a lack of incentive for hospitals' preparatory efforts, there is no mandate requiring such activity. Currently, the closest thing to a hospital mandate is a Joint Commission on the Accreditation of Health Care Organizations (JCAHO) requirement that every hospital have emergency plans and drills in place to cover a broad range of potential disasters.

Legal mandates and financial incentives will likely be required to catalyze hospital response on this issue. At least four types of financial protection will be necessary:

- Funds to help hospitals address fundamental capacity and infrastructure deficiencies,
- Funds for outbreak response planning and preparedness,
- Compensation for direct patient care in the event of an outbreak, combined with a loosening of the usual requirements for detailed corroborating documentation, and
- Reimbursement for extraordinary institutional costs.

In addition, immunity from liability will be necessary in the context of actions that outbreak management typically entails: triage decisions, dealing with immuno-suppressed populations, mandatory vaccination, and quarantine.

Regional Collaborative Networks

An effective community response to an outbreak will require that multiple health organizations and the public and private sectors respond in a highly integrated fashion. This collaboration must bridge at least three distinct health communities—public health, emergency management/first responders, and medical care delivery—each of which has its own culture, language, and decision-making processes. All three communities will need to be linked with local and state elected and government authorities, law and order institutions, state laboratories, military hospitals, the Centers for Disease Control and Prevention (CDC), and other agencies.

However, substantial communications and knowledge barriers exist within and among all of these various health agencies. For example, a recent TOPOFF exercise, named for its engagement of top officials of the U.S. government, was held in Denver in spring 2000. It tested the readiness of government officials and agencies to respond to a bioweapons event. In an assessment of TOPOFF, a number of the participants noted that different professions practiced different decision-making processes. One observer commented that, "In public health, most decision-making is through democratic processes and consensus-building, but for some decisions, this cannot work." Another observer remarked, "The time frame that public health is accustomed to dealing with is not what is needed for bioterrorism. In this type of crisis, one needs to make decisions quickly. You don't have the luxury of time to do more research." One public health official noted a widespread lack of familiarity with terms—such as a JIC (Joint Information Center), a JOC (Joint Operations Center), or DMORTs (Disaster Mortuary Assistance Teams)—used by the emergency management community (Inglesby et al., 2001).

As another example of a communications barrier, during the West Nile outbreak in New York City in 1999, an infectious disease physician from one of the boroughs notified the New York City Department of Health about two suspected cases of encephalitis. In the meantime, 20 other patients with encephalitis had already been admitted to other NYC hospitals. Although encephalitis is clearly recognizable and is considered a legally reportable disease in New York, none of those other 20 cases had been called in (O'Toole, 2000). Even if these cases had been called in, the capacity of the health agency to respond adequately is uncertain. Dr. John Bartlett, Chief of Infectious Disease at Johns Hopkins University School of Medicine, conducted an experiment two years ago in the Hopkins emergency department, during which he simulated a patient with a case of inhalational anthrax. During this exercise, which occurred during a summer weekend, no one he contacted either inside or outside the Hopkins hospital was certain about which telephone number to use or which state official to notify (Osterholm and Schwartz, 2000). Finally, a call was made to the state public health officer and an urgent message left on an answering machine. Due to a lack of beepers in the public health department, the call was not answered until three days later.

Although the federal government has initiated efforts to create linkages among the emergency management and public health services in 50 to 60 cities nationwide, no region has yet truly integrated emergency management, public health, and medical services. An effective regional network requires adequate funding, designation of an in-charge organization and individual, and development of a regional response plan that would need to be rehearsed, critiqued, and modified as appropriate. Among the many challenges to overcome are the climate of competition among hospitals, distrust across the public-/private-sector divide, and communications and cultural obstacles among the multiple health communities.

Staffing and Legal/Policy Issues

Several groups of hospital executives have assembled over the past year under the auspices of the Johns Hopkins Center for Civilian Biodefense and the American Hospital Association (supported by the Department of Health and Human Services' [DHHS'] Office of Emergency Preparedness). Their objective has been to identify issues and barriers to hospitals' response to bioterrorism. One set of concerns pertains to hospital staffing, specifically:

- Staff shortages, which cut across multiple professional and non-professional categories, are national in scope (in the case of nursing, international) and, given declines in academic enrollments for some professions, will likely be long-lasting.
- For many health care professions (including physicians, nurses, and pharmacists), licensing restrictions prohibit individuals from practicing across state borders. If unaddressed, this will act as a barrier to importing physicians and nurses from outside crisis areas.
- Seventy to eighty percent of hospital staff are female, the majority of whom are heads of households or are responsible for the care of family members. In the event of a major epidemic, which could last for weeks or months, the issue of family support becomes critical (Bentley, 2000).
- Personal protection in the form of immunizations and access to antibiotics for staff and their families is a critical issue. It is unclear how

health care staff will respond to future outbreaks, though it may be instructive to look back at workers' and professionals' concerns during the early days of the AIDS epidemic.

A second set of concerns pertains to legal issues. For example, the Emergency Medical Treatment and Labor Act (EMTALA) was designed to prohibit hospitals from refusing treatment to uninsured patients and sending them to other hospitals. The legislation requires each hospital to screen and stabilize every patient, even during a disease outbreak when it is likely that a hospital's emergency room may be closed for containment purposes. Also, different hospitals may have different roles in a public health emergency; for example, some may be used solely for quarantine, others for triage, and still others for specialized treatment. Thus, during an outbreak, not all hospitals may be capable of screening and stabilizing every patient. The EMTALA was not designed with an era of emerging infections in mind (Bentley, 2000).

EMTALA may be just the tip of the iceberg of unresolved legal and public policy issues, many of which relate to the fragmented U.S. legal system. For example, the legal powers that authorize response in a public health emergency are divided between the national and local levels. Interestingly, legal power may depend on whether an epidemic is deemed to be natural or intentional; national security law might apply in the case of the latter (Fidler, 2000).

A legal system that emphasizes protection of individual rights, while restricting government powers from impinging on such rights, creates additional potential barriers to an effective public health response. For example, citizens might ignore government orders, such as travel bans, quarantine, or compulsory treatment directives, which could, in turn, increase the likelihood that military intervention would be necessary to enforce public health (Fidler, 2000).

Conclusion

It would be inappropriate to conclude without putting into a larger context the challenge of preparing our health care system to respond to future epidemics. As previously mentioned, there may be legitimate conflicting perspectives on what role the health care system should assume in the event of a major public health crisis. These perspectives are buttressed by age-old differences in skill sets and attitudes between the medical and public health disciplines, and by large cultural gaps between triage and treatment, containment and continuous quality improvement, and isolation and architectural openness. A Stanford University Hospital analysis found that the routine hospitalized patient encounters over 30 different hospital employees during an average 24-hour period—hardly an ideal environment from which to try to contain an epidemic. Nonetheless, hospitals can and should play a major role in outbreak response:

- The population will undoubtedly continue to seek hospital care for diagnosis, treatment, and prophylaxis. The absence of treatment facilities could contribute to public panic.
- Hospitals are socially and geographically well-established arsenals within their communities, constituting well-known loci where professionals, equipment, supplies, and information technology come together in the service of local communities.

However, it is remarkable how quickly local hospital capacity is overwhelmed in many, if not all, epidemic-response scenarios. There is a need for sophisticated modeling of a range of hypothetical outbreaks, using current hospital capacity data. More importantly, we should explore all reasonable mechanisms to help hospitals substantially expand their capacities to handle mass surges of people (by incremental hundreds or even thousands) in the event of a major epidemic. One option, for example, might be to create expandable bio-containment units, which would be self-contained but placed adjacent to hospitals. Such units might enable the use of the existing hospitals' organizational infrastructures, supplies, and personnel, while providing a simple but epidemiologically sound setting for the triage and treatment of far more individuals than the institutions' emergency rooms or clinics could safely handle. Similarly, we might explore the feasibility of training a cadre of hospital-based epidemiologists, current EMS physicians, and new staff. These suggestions and speculations are offered as a point of departure for future discussions on how best to help America's health care system prepare for inevitable disease outbreaks.

VACCINES FOR POST-ELIMINATION CONTINGENCIES

Thomas P. Monath, M.D.

Vice President, Research and Medical Affairs
Acambis Inc., Cambridge, MA

Vaccines have been by far the most efficient means to prevent and control infectious diseases. Smallpox eradication was achieved through vaccination, and the eradication of poliovirus and measles will be achieved when the prevalence of artificial immunity is sufficiently high to preclude interhuman transmission. The benefits of disease eradication achieved through vaccination include life years gained; savings to patients, families, and society due to reduced morbidity and mortality; avoidance of costs for treatment and continued vaccination; indirect cost savings due to increased productivity; and the freeing-up of health care resources for other interventions. Following successful eradication, a responsible policy must include provisions for vaccine reserves and contingency planning in case the disease re-emerges; surveillance and diagnostic activities; and research on and development of new vaccines and therapeutic drugs.

Rationale for Vaccine Reserves

Because surveillance and case-finding may be difficult, particularly in medically underserved regions, disease eradication may be uncertain for several years after the last reported case. During this period of watchfulness, rumors of disease and case and outbreak investigations will continue, and vaccine must be available in the event of re-emergence. The means by which a disease could be reintroduced after presumptive elimination are listed in Table 6-1. For smallpox and other diseases under consideration for potential elimination—polio, measles, and rubella—no enzootic or nonhuman reservoir has been identified as a source of reintroduction; thus, the principal risks are human factors, inadvertent escape of laboratory stocks, and intentional release (bioterrorism or biowarfare). The consequences of reintroduction become increasingly grave over time due to the decline of herd immunity, susceptibility of the population to a pandemic, senescence of surveillance and laboratory diagnostic capability, and reduced medical awareness.

Smallpox as a Case Study

When smallpox was eradicated in 1979, re-emergence was dismissed as highly unlikely for several reasons:

TABLE 6-1 Sources of Disease Re-Emergence After Eradication

- Chronic infection and reactivation (e.g., immunosuppressed hosts)
- Natural reservoir or zoonotic cycle
- Closely-related agent fills niche of original virus
- Vaccine manufacturer's seed viruses
- Research laboratory stocks
- Stored diagnostic specimens
- Cross-contaminated or mislabeled laboratory materials
- Environmental sources, fomites, human remains (e.g., permafrost)
- Biological weapons, surreptitious stocks, accidents, weapons tests, intentional releases

- There was no enzootic reservoir; monkeypox and other zoonotic poxviruses related to the smallpox virus were not considered a significant source for the reintroduction of human pox virus.
- There were only a limited number of laboratories working with smallpox, and confidence was high that all laboratory stocks had been identified and destroyed. Reference materials were deposited in only two laboratories, one in the United States and the other in the Soviet Union.
- There was no evidence that smallpox virus could persist or be reactivated in previously infected humans.
- There was a high degree of confidence that vaccine reserves (approximately 200 million doses deposited at WHO) were adequate for any contingency and vaccine manufacture could be reinstated if necessary.
- There was little concern about any threat posed by biowarfare (BW).

In the United States, vaccine manufacture ceased in 1982, and immunization of soldiers ceased in 1989 (Table 6-2).

Smallpox was dismissed as a bioweapon in part because all countries, including the USSR, had participated actively in eradication of the disease. It was, therefore, a surprise to learn that the Soviet Union, a nation engaged in the eradication effort, would simultaneously engage in surreptitious, state-sanctioned activities that could result in disease reintroduction. Moreover, smallpox has undesirable features as a bioweapon for several reasons: the disease is easily diagnosed; attribution of an attack would be obvious; the virus is transmissible and could backfire on non-target populations; the incubation period is long and its effect on a target population delayed; and a vaccine is available and routinely used to protect military forces.

The fallacy of these conclusions was not apparent until the early 1990s, after a defector from the former USSR revealed that smallpox was considered a strategic (not tactical) weapon. Development of smallpox as a BW

TABLE 6-2 Smallpox Vaccination History, United States

1949	Last indigenous cases of smallpox (Texas)
1969–1970	Studies emphasize high incidence of vaccine-related adverse events
1971–1972	Routine vaccination of children ceases
1976	Vaccination of medical workers ceases
1979	Eradication certified by WHO
1982	Wyeth ceases vaccine manufacture
1989	U.S. military ceases vaccination of soldiers
2000	Over half the U.S. population unvaccinated Vulnerability to pandemic spread if reintroduced

TABLE 6-3 Vaccine Policy After Smallpox Eradication

1980–1997
- Need for vaccine considered very remote
- No requirement for continued manufacture
- Reliance on stocks of final filled containers

1998–2000
- Need for vaccine considered urgent (bioterrorism)
- Vaccine reserves diminished due to stability problems
- Requirement for continuous manufacture recognized
- New regulatory requirements for modernized vaccine
- Government procurement process initiated (1999)
- Manufacturer contracted (2000)
- Time to new stockpile of licensed vaccine: Five years

agent had begun shortly after World War II, and the virus had been fully deployed in strategic weapons (Alibek, 1999). Intelligence leaks suggested that countries other than the former USSR were investigating smallpox as a BW agent as well, and by 1998, smallpox was widely considered the preferred biological weapon for terrorist activities (Henderson et al., 1999). By this time, it was recognized that U.S. vulnerability was enhanced by a deficient vaccine reserve since no vaccine had been produced since 1982, and the remaining static stockpile had partially deteriorated (LeDuc and Becher, 1999). The result was a complete shift in the policy for vaccine reserves within the public health sector (Table 6-3). In September 2000, the Centers for Disease Control and Prevention issued a contract to Acambis, Inc. (formerly known as OraVax, Inc.) for manufacture of a national stockpile of 40 million doses of a modern cell culture vaccine approved for use by the U.S. Food and Drug Administration (FDA).

Meanwhile, motivated by the hypothetical BW threat, the deteriorating vaccine reserves, and unacceptable characteristics of the original calf-lymph vaccine, the U.S. military had reinstated a vaccine development program in 1988. Its original objective was to produce a new cell culture-derived vaccine that could be administered by parenteral injection (thus avoiding the local cutaneous lesion responsible for auto- and accidental inoculation). Although some headway was made over the following twelve years and three small clinical trials conducted, the military program did not advance beyond pilot lot manufacture and investigational status, and it did not address the larger public health concerns.

Bioterrorism and Vaccine Reserves

These events emphasize how the changing landscape following disease eradication affects vaccine policies. The threat of deliberate release will remain the most significant rationale for a responsible and conservative policy. Measles, a highly infectious agent that would cause significant morbidity in non-immune adult populations, is another potential BW agent. Even poliovirus, which is far less transmissible and has a high infection:case ratio, should not be dismissed. The pathogenesis of poliovirus delivered as an aerosol could be fundamentally different from that of the naturally occurring disease.

The size of a vaccine reserve after elimination of these diseases must be carefully considered. The stockpile should be disease-specific and dependent on the prevalence of immunity required to break transmission. Transmission dynamic modeling may be useful in determining the size of the vaccine reserve. In the case of smallpox, limited data from the pre-vaccine era may provide a baseline for prediction. For measles, data on outbreaks in developing country populations with very low immunization coverage could be used. Similarily, polio outbreaks prior to the introduction of vaccine could provide data from which the spread of the the disease in an unprotected population may be modelled. While these examples may not offer exact models, they provide some basis for estimating the potential impact of outbreaks in the post-eradication era and thus, an appropriate size of a vaccine reserve.

Rationale for Continued Manufacture, Research, and Development

In retrospect, the decision to terminate smallpox vaccine manufacture, research, and development at the time of disease eradication and, instead, rely on existing stocks of vaccine to meet emergent contingencies was fallacious. The political, regulatory (i.e., regulatory requirements pertaining to vaccine safety), and scientific (e.g., genetic modifications to the disease agent) landscapes are expected to change significantly over time after elimination of any infectious disease agent. These changes require a supply of in-date vaccine, combined with continued vaccine research and development.

As examples of changing regulatory requirements, several unforeseen safety issues have arisen within the last decade:

- The risk of prion-mediated diseases resulting from the incorporation of bovine and human derivatives (fetal calf serum, human serum albumin, gelatin, and lactose) into vaccines.
- Concern about mercury, which has resulted in the removal of thimerosol from vaccines.
- Concern about adventitious agents, which has resulted in new quality control tests, including assays to detect replication-competent retroviruses and new standards for residuals (in particular, DNA). For example, in the case of smallpox vaccine, the static stockpile preserved at the time of

eradication was produced in bovine tissue from individual animals that had not been tested for adventitious agents. Given the popular concerns about vaccine safety, it is easy to imagine the outcry of concern if the smallpox vaccine stockpile were to be activated.

Vaccine Manufacture After Disease Elimination

To ensure an adequate supply of vaccine that meets current good manufacturing practices requirements, at least one U.S. manufacturer of the vaccine in question should maintain active production and testing after disease eradication. This would require that master and working seed viruses be periodically tested under a formal stability program, and that the volume and number of containers of working seed are adequate to meet contingencies for scaled-up production. Since bulk can be stored for longer periods than final containers, a large supply of bulk vaccine should be kept frozen and ready for filling and finishing, although the filled vaccine stockpile must be sufficient to meet emergency requirements. As noted previously, the number of vials stored for this purpose will be determined by transmission modeling based on a worst-case scenario. New bulk vaccine and filled containers will be replenished on a schedule determined by stability data; expertise and experience of the corporate manufacturing and control personnel will be maintained; and the facilities, equipment, production process, and quality control methods will be continually validated. The Biologics License should be maintained, and regulatory staff (at FDA) should remain familiar with the product. By following these guidelines, the capability for surge production will be ensured.

Change from profitable to orphan product

Elimination of the disease will have a profound effect on the commercial status of the respective vaccine(s). In particular, vaccine status will change from large-volume, profit-driven markets to an orphan product. Large-scale continuous production will need to be modified in order to meet the demands of the new, smaller scale of the vaccine reserve program, which might entail campaigned production in shared facilities. This smaller scale will undoubtedly increase unit dose costs. Moreover, new security requirements will need to be imposed to protect seeds and vaccine, and biocontainment levels may increase in order to prevent escape of the virus from the facilities. These changes are likely to make the vaccine reserve program less profitable and more troublesome, with the result that the original manufacturer(s), typically large pharmaceutical companies, may lose interest. Therefore, it will be necessary to supplant commercial sales with a government supply contract. If smaller, "hungrier" biopharmaceutical companies become engaged in the government-sponsored vaccine production, a period of technology transfer, process validation, and possibly bridging clinical trials, may be required. Technology transfer requires infrastructure and expertise and may take several years (or longer) to accomplish.

Vaccine stability

Vaccine stability is the key factor in determining the scale and schedule of vaccine reserve manufacture. Stability is both vaccine- and virus-specific, as well as temperature-dependent. Bulk vaccine can be stored for considerably longer than can final, filled containers. For example, polio and measles vaccine bulks can be stored frozen for ten years, whereas final filled containers of measles and inactivated polio vaccines have shelf lives of two and three years, respectively. Real-time stability studies are necessary to establish expiration dating and would need to be repeated if vaccine manufacturing were transferred from one company to another.

Surge capacity

A key element in planning for post-elimination contingencies is the capacity of the vaccine manufacturer to scale-up production without changing the validated manufacturing process. The primary response to an emergency would involve using stored bulk vaccine to produce filled vials. However, it should be noted that approximately three months are required to fill vaccine and complete release tests. Seed stocks and cell banks must be available in sufficient supply. Manufacturing could be expanded by simply increasing the number of bioreactors (production vessels) and production suites. However, surge manufacturing must conform to validated processes so that no new regulatory problems arise. Production scale could be modestly increased (e.g., tenfold) without significantly changing the manufacturing process, although it is advised that the scaled-up process be tested and validated in advance.

New distribution requirements

In the post-elimination era, the fundamental approach to vaccine distribution will change, from routine childhood immunization programs to emergency mass immunization campaigns. In lieu of direct sales to private physicians, sales through physician supply houses, and local health department routine immunization programs, the federal government will prepare to distribute vaccine in the context of an emergency program. The storage and distribution system must be consistent with federal emergency planning, and packaging and labeling must be consistent with the intended use under emergency conditions. Methods for rapid large-scale vaccine administration must also be considered, since safety concerns preclude use of the multi-dose jet-injector. If new devices replace the original jet-injector, it will be necessary to conduct clinical trials with the reserve vaccine(s) to demonstrate immunogenicity.

Vaccine liability

After disease elimination, the vaccine status under the National Vaccine Injury Compensation Program would change, since the program currently applies only to routine pediatric vaccines. In the case of smallpox vaccine, which was never covered by the program, the manufacturer (Acambis, Inc.) contracted by CDC to produce new vaccine in response to bioterrorism threats was required to indemnify the government against tort claims. This was especially difficult because of the relatively high incidence of serious adverse events expected with widespread vaccine usage. Private insurance was obtained at a high cost to the government. A more cost-effective alternative would be to amend the Public Health Service Act so the government could indemnify the manufacturer.

Re-Initiating or Changing Vaccine Production

Since biological products cannot be characterized as discrete, single-component chemical structures, they are controlled primarily by demonstrating consistency of manufacturing. Changes to the manufacturing process or vaccine composition, which may affect vaccine performance, require significant effort in terms of validation and clinical testing. Old vaccines that undergo such changes are considered new vaccines by the regulatory authority, and new requirements not applicable under grandfather approvals may be imposed. Examples include: 1) programs for redevelopment after lapsed production (e.g., vaccinia virus formerly made by Wyeth and now redeveloped by Acambis); 2) modernization of the vaccine manufacturing process and facilities (e.g., anthrax vaccine formerly made by Michigan State Laboratories and now by Bioport); and 3) transfer of manufacturing (e.g., influenza from Parke-Davis to King Pharmaceutics, and yellow fever vaccine from Wellcome to Evans Vaccines). Each of these cases required a considerable, lengthy effort. For example, Acambis' accelerated vaccinia production will require approximately five years from project initiation to establishment of a new national vaccine stockpile. Problems associated with changes in the manufacturing process should be anticipated in the event that old vaccines, such as polio, are transitioned from routine use to a vaccine reserve status.

Vaccine Research and Development After Disease Elimination

After a disease has been eliminated, the natural tendency is to reduce both public and private funding for research and development. This causes a rapid erosion of technical expertise and capabilities to meet new and unforeseen contingencies. In the case of smallpox, this erosion was mitigated by the use of vaccinia as a live vector for vaccines and gene therapy. However, it is unlikely that polio and measles virus expertise will be maintained after eradication without a dedicated effort. Future threats may require modifications to the antigenic profile of vaccines; new studies on the immunological basis for protection; and the ability of vaccines to protect against strains having altered pathogenesis or route of infection. To meet these needs, a strong federally-sponsored research program must be maintained.

STRATEGIC PRIORITIES FOR ADDRESSING POST-ERADICATION OUTBREAKS

Robert P. Kadlec, M.D.

Colonel, U.S. Air Force and Professor
Military Strategy and Operations
National War College, National Defense University
Washington, D.C.

The eradication of globally significant diseases is properly entrusted to the public health and medical communities. However, the long-term implications of such efforts, including the possibility of natural or deliberate post-eradication outbreaks, may have security as well as public health consequences. The possible security implications of disease eradication should be assessed at the outset. This involves determining what, if any, bioterrorism, biological warfare or serious epidemic risk the agent represents and what steps should be taken to minimize those risks.

Five strategic priorities that should be addressed in a post-eradication outbreak are:

1. recognize that it is occurring;
2. contain its possible spread and mitigate its effects;
3. characterize it;
4. if possible, prevent its recurrence; and,
5. if necessary, hold those responsible accountable.

Since the last documented endemic case of smallpox in 1977, the only other known occurrence was limited to a laboratory accident in 1978. The smallpox success story, however, illustrates the possible paradoxical security outcome of viral eradication. While the natural occurrence of this disease is a distant memory, the prospect of a deliberate post-eradication outbreak as the result of a terrorist attack or act of war is now considered credible. The non-immune status of the majority of Americans, coupled with a limited national capacity to respond to an outbreak, leaves a significant vulnerability which terrorists or adversaries could threaten to exploit.

The later stages of the public health effort to eradicate smallpox were not effectively synchronized or coordinated with the Department of Defense (DoD) attempt to assess the national security implications of the overall effort. This asynchrony left several notable shortfalls. The U.S. government did not invest in the preservation of capacities to produce and maintain adequate supplies of smallpox vaccine; it did not ensure the development of appropriate diagnostics; and it did not conduct research into antiviral therapies or assess the efficacy of existing vaccine to counter a smallpox biowarfare or terrorist threat. These issues contributed to the U.S. policy decision to delay the ultimate destruction of the remaining known smallpox cultures.

Eradication-Associated Security Assessment

Without careful consideration, the successful eradication of other diseases could result in similar scenarios, where the suspension of immunization practices and loss of vaccine production capabilities could lead to increased public health vulnerability and possible national security consequences. Prudent public health and national security policies require a formal assessment process to determine if eradication could lead to such a paradoxical security outcome. Central to this assessment is consideration of a possible natural or deliberate post-eradication outbreak. Eradication is a public health and medical responsibility, but assessing the possible security implications is a multidisciplinary process involving several non-health participants—including intelligence, arms control, law enforcement, and defense communities—whose roles would be distinct from but supportive of the actual eradication process.

The fundamental question to answer in an eradication-associated security assessment is, what is the disease's biowarfare and epidemic potential? Most of the information needed to answer this question should already be available. Factors that need to be considered include disease virulence, transmissibility, environmental stability, and the availability of diagnostics, prophylaxis, and treatment. Infectious agents that lend themselves to biowarfare or bioterrorism should receive greater security scrutiny than ones that do not in an effort to narrow the list of agents requiring further review, contingency planning, and possible resource investment.

Intelligence and Arms Control Issues

If the disease agent has biowarfare potential, its inclusion in formal biological arms control negotiations could be a logical next step. A legally binding protocol to the Biological Weapons and Toxins Convention (BWTC), which is currently being negotiated, may include provisions that take into account disease eradication efforts. It may be possible and desirable to give special prohibited status to eradicated diseases. The nature of the prohibitions, and possible consequences for violating such provisions, would be determined largely by the terms of the eradication agreement and the nature of the disease agent. Linking the arms control process with the eradication effort combines the formal legally and politically binding commitments of a multilateral arms control treaty with the moral commitment of a public health action.

Verification and transparency are additional arms control concepts worth considering during disease eradication efforts. Verification is a formal, legally binding certification mechanism between participating parties. It is the process one uses to ascertain the compliance of parties with an agreement, and it represents the confidence one has about that compliance. It also serves as a potential incentive for compliance. For the purposes of eradication, the verification process could assist in determining, with a high level of certainty, whether a disease has been eliminated from all natural reservoirs and been accounted for in laboratories and all other possible repositories.

Arms control verification can never be 100%. It may, however, serve as a useful theoretical framework and possible metric when considering possible security implications. For example, if one's verification process is strong and confidence in verification high, possible security issues are different than if the process were weak and confidence low. Historically, biological arms control verification has been considered problematic, if not impossible. Microbial agents, equipment, and processes to produce them can be used for both peaceful as well as prohibited uses. The dual-use nature of microbial research, development, and production are considered major impediments to achieving effective verification. Instead, biological arms control promotes the concept of transparency that provides openness about certain activities, like biodefense for example, that could be matters of concern but refrains from making any formal treaty determination about those activities. Transparency of only selected activities can build confidence in compliance while implicitly acknowledging the inherent limits of and low confidence about verification.

Intelligence and arms control issues should be considered and addressed appropriately. The intelligence community has the ability to collect and assess information that can help determine whether the disease agent in question has biowarfare potential or has been researched or developed as such, and whether nations or groups may seek to develop that agent as a weapon. Most importantly, intelligence can assist in assessing compliance with the terms of the effort. By collecting all source information, they may be able to determine whether the intent of participating parties is consistent with their overt actions. Thus, their involvement is vital to helping establish a level of confidence in compliance with the eradication process.

Department of Defense's Role in the Eradication Process

The DoD has both the clinical and laboratory resources to play several possible roles in the eradication process. For example, as part of theater engagement plans, military medical units provide medical support and assistance, including vaccination, to developing nations on an on-going basis. Similarly, several overseas military laboratories offer regional laboratory expertise that can, and has, supported eradication efforts.

The DoD is responsible for assessing the potential impact of eradication campaigns on the future health and operational effectiveness of U.S. military personnel. Immunizations are administered either upon entry into the armed forces or prior to deployments into areas where endemic or biowarfare threats are considered significant. While the natural foci of disease may be eliminated, suspension of immunizations for active and reserve military personnel follow a different set of priorities than in the civilian sector. The nature of the disease and its potential operational impact must be considered, as well as any and all intelligence that may provide insight into adversaries' intentions or capabilities to use the agent for biowarfare purposes.

The military's need to protect its troops goes beyond vaccines; it also involves diagnostic capabilities, possible biodetection technologies, chemoprophylaxis, and therapeutics. The military has an obligation to engage early in the eradication process. A security review offers an opportunity to assess what capabilities are needed to protect America's armed forces from future threats.

With the current concern about bioterrorism and asymmetric warfare, the public health community may find the defense approach to threat assessment and capabilities development relevant. If the agent subject to eradication is deemed to be of biowarfare or serious epidemic potential, the DoD's requirements for diagnostics, detection technologies, vaccines, and prophylactics may also be applicable. From a public health perspective, it may also be valuable to conduct age-stratified longitudinal studies to assess and monitor the changing status of the population's immunity. Over time, the population's immune status may become an indicator of vulnerability, which may help guide policy-making and later resource allocation.

Planning for Future Security Risks

Once it has been determined that a disease may have future security implications, the five priorities cited earlier become the functional basis for planning. Recognizing a possible post-eradication outbreak is the first and foremost priority. An extensive, interconnected global and national surveillance and laboratory system must be able to recognize and confirm the event. The sentinels of this system, however, are health care workers. While a disease may be eradicated, there may still be a need to ensure that primary care providers have sufficient clinical knowledge and index of suspicion about the disease to include it in their differential diagnosis. To this end, laboratory diagnostics that can confirm the diagnosis must be available.

Following immediate recognition, a prompt response is necessary to contain and mitigate the outbreak's morbidity and mortality. Depending on the agent, an international response may be required to augment individual national capabilities, as well as address the possible risk of regional or global spread. Vaccines and other products may be required. Stockpiles, pharmaceutical surge capacities, and logistics to move these supplies will determine the timeliness and effectiveness of the response.

Outbreak characterization and containment should occur simultaneously. In addition to traditional "shoe leather" and molecular epidemiology, other types of information, including intelligence sources, may be required to help determine whether the outbreak was a natural occurrence, suspicious, or deliberate. If suspicious or deliberate, there may be a requirement to collect evidence for legal or arms control purposes. Prevention of recurrence is largely dependent on the results of epidemiological and other investigations. Finally, holding responsible parties accountable may depend on the outcome of arms control, law enforcement, and even intelligence investigations. The response to a deliberate outbreak falls into the domain of political and possible legal action beyond the scope of this discussion.

Security Issues Related to Measles Eradication

The case of measles offers a brief illustration of the range of possible security issues related to disease eradication. Measles is an infectious disease agent that offers a realistic target for future eradication: humans are the only natural host for wild-type measles virus; an effective measles vaccine is available; following immunization, immunity to natural infection is long-lived; accurate diagnostic tests are available; and recent regional efforts have demonstrated success in interrupting measles transmission in the United States and Western Hemisphere.

Should a concerted effort be initiated to achieve global eradication, a first step in assessing the possible security implications would be to assess the biowarfare potential of measles. Measles is transmitted by respiratory droplets and is highly contagious. It can remain infective in droplet form in air for several hours, especially in low relative humidity (CDC, 1992), and can be transmitted by airborne spread as aerosolized droplet nuclei. Under these conditions, it is possible that a biowarfare aerosol release of measles virus could result in infection in exposed, non-immune individuals. Measles causes significant morbidity and mortality in children and is even more severe in adults. In one study, 30% of adult cases exhibited bacterial superinfection of the respiratory tract, 17% exhibited evidence of bronchospasm, and 3% developed pneumonia requiring hospitalization (Gremillion and Crawford, 1981).

The biowarfare potential of measles would probably figure prominently into the defense community's assessment of measles elimination. Given the likelihood of significant complications in military-age populations and the possibility of natural or other reservoirs, future DoD vaccination policies would probably have to take into account possible post-eradication outbreaks.

Properly administered measles vaccine results in immunity lasting for at least 16 years (Markowitz and Katz, 1994), but possible security concerns may require further longitudinal studies evaluating the duration of vaccine-induced immunity. Even if civilian vaccine practices were curtailed or discontinued, it may still be necessary to immunize the military or at least maintain a stockpile of measles vaccine, which would require planning and budgeting for an uninterrupted or standby surge production capacity. If the biowarfare threat from measles were deemed credible, the efficacy of the current vaccine might have to be assessed in the context of aerosolized transmission, which would depend on identifying an appropriate animal model for human measles. If researchers found that the vaccine were not entirely protective, research into possible antiviral therapies may be warranted. Surveillance systems would have to be geared to meet a possible measles threat, and rapid clinical diagnostics and detector technologies may have to be researched and developed. These are only a few of the possible issues that may have to be addressed during a security-based review.

Conclusion

Incorporating a national security process into an eradication effort introduces a dimension not commonly encountered in public health debates. On the one hand, it involves activities that strengthen the objective and purpose of the eradication effort. On the other hand, it raises concerns that may be new to public health practitioners. Security reviews may alter the public health community's fundamental expectations for eradication, and raise questions about traditional assumptions concerning disease eradication. For example, the conventional wisdom associating significant financial savings with ending routine immunizations may be challenged. Money saved on immunizations may have to be spent on expanded surveillance and vaccine stockpiling programs, for example. As America enters the 21st century, cognizant of the revolutions in biotechnology and genetics and the prospect of biowarfare, the health and security communities must work together to ensure both public health and national security. Disease eradication supports both imperatives, but the long-term consequences must be anticipated from the outset.

UNDERSTANDING THE PUBLIC AND MEDIA RESPONSE TO AN OUTBREAK

Ann E. Norwood, M.D.

Colonel, U.S. Army Medical Corps
Associate Professor and Associate Chair, Department of Psychiatry
Uniformed Services University of the Health Sciences, Bethesda, MD

A swift, well-coordinated, and effective public health response is the most powerful psychological intervention in a post-eradication outbreak. Through their actions and comments, political leaders, public health experts, and other key figures at the local, state, and federal levels will shape individual and community expectations, beliefs, and behaviors. In particular, the management of the outbreak in the first hours to days sets the tone for societal responses.

Fear and the Public Reaction

Infection by a microorganism taps into very deep-rooted fears of being invaded and destroyed by an invisible force. The lack of sensory cues associated with infection makes it impossible to discern whether or not one has been infected. Many organisms produce ubiquitous symptoms that can go undiagnosed until it is too late to save the victim. A delayed onset between exposure and illness produces tremendous anxiety and uncertainty in those fearing they have been infected. Moreover, much of the public does not have the scientific background with which to understand the outbreak.

By definition, post-eradication outbreaks would produce diseases rarely seen in medical practice. There would be limited medical knowledge about diagnosis, treatment, and outcome in the general community. This poses considerable uncertainty for both physicians and patients. In many countries, an epidemic of a disease that produces a high acute mortality rate will be a new experience. While people can become accustomed to quite terrible circumstances, there is a great possibility of panic when they are exposed to an unfamiliar threat for the first time. For example, the first use of gas and the introduction of machine guns in war both produced panic in the troops. As soldiers became familiar with these weapons, however, panic dissipated. Exposure to the dead and disfigured also produces strong psychological responses and is a potent psychological stressor.

Understanding which aspects of biological agents invoke terror can aid in developing intervention strategies. For example, unrealistic beliefs about microbes and viruses can be addressed through education. Informing people about what they can expect, thereby lessening surprise and affording them a sense of control through predictability, can alleviate uncertainty.

Fear-producing aspects of outbreaks include:

- the potential for high numbers of casualties;
- a potentially limited availability of treatments;
- in some cases, uncertainty about the effectiveness of medical interventions;
- the possibility of an epidemic involving person-to-person transmission; and
- dispersion of the ill, which can erode the sense of safety in regions far from the original source of infection.

Based on data gleaned from studies of disasters and observations of past outbreaks, there are certain elements of an outbreak that influence the public's reaction. How an outbreak has arisen has major implications for behaviors. An act of bioterrorism, for example, can be expected to provoke widespread rage which can be difficult to manage with respect to scapegoating. It could also result in ill-advised policy decisions made in the heat of the moment. Grotesqueness has been demonstrated to be a powerful predictor of strong emotional responses. Diseases like smallpox and hemorrhagic fevers, such as Ebola, evoke terror in many people. The larger the outbreak, the more strain it places on the community. The disruption of basic community functions and normal activities adds secondary psychological and behavioral stressors.

The media will play a major role in determining how the public reacts following an outbreak. In a climate of uncertainty and fear, the public will thirst for information to help them gauge their personal risks. Radio, television, and the Internet should be used to provide accurate, non-sensationalized information in order to control rumors and provide instructions on personal safety measures.

Psychological responses to outbreaks of eradicated disease can include:

the attribution of somatic symptoms to intoxication and infection, scapegoating and stigmatization, and social isolation and paranoia, which contribute to the development of conspiracy theories and mistrust. As the outbreak continues, people may become demoralized and lose their faith in the institutions that are supposed to protect them. All of these responses are influenced by cultural and religious views about causality, death, and dying. Therefore, it is very difficult to generalize findings across cultures and over time.

The Nature of Panic

The word "panic" is often used to describe psychological responses to disease outbreaks. Panic refers primarily to a group phenomenon in which intense, contagious fear causes individuals to think only of themselves. They become paralyzed by fear or seek to escape by any means necessary. Panic also refers to an individual response characterized by the loss of rational thought due to overwhelming terror. A major goal of preparation and response for a post-eradication outbreak is the prevention of panic and the preservation of individual, group, and community function.

In examining historical responses to epidemics, Garrett (1994) has made the following observations:

> Panic does not always go hand in hand with epidemics, nor does its scale correlate with the general gravity of the situation. Indeed, history demonstrates that population responses to diseases are rarely predictable, often peculiar. . . . Where a hefty dose of public concern was warranted, as in the case of the 1918–19 [influenza] pandemic, an oddly common feature was nonchalance. . . . In contrast, public reaction to the 29 deaths in Philadelphia [Legionnaires' disease] was extraordinary. . . . Phrases like "explosive outbreak," "mysterious and terrifying disease," "Legionnaire killer," and "killer pneumonia" filled press accounts as well as the on-camera statements of Philadelphians and politicians.

As this statement implies, the way the news is covered shapes the public response to an outbreak.

Panic is rare following disasters. For example, panic did not occur following the Tokyo sarin attack; although thousands of people sought medical care after the sarin attack, they were orderly and obeyed instructions, and first responders and hospital staff managed their responsibilities well. However, this may not happen during an epidemic. The risk factors for panic are:

- surprise and novelty,
- the belief that there is only a small chance of escape,
- seeing oneself as high risk for becoming ill,

- available, but limited, resources in which there is a situation of "first come, first served,"
- a perceived lack of effective management of the catastrophe, and
- loss of credibility of authorities.

The government and medical community will play large roles in shaping the public's reaction. Medical responses will be scrutinized for efficacy and fairness. For example, political and medical decisions about what groups to vaccinate first, or which groups will be given highest priority for a limited supply of vaccine, may have a chilling effect. These decisions may also affect those responsible for providing medical care and other essential community services. For example, a question that frequently arises in the first responder community is, "In the event of a contagious agent, would our families be given high priority as well as us?" Policy makers must address how decisions in this area will be made and explained to the public. Protocols should be developed for these scenarios in order to mitigate panic and minimize the risk of poor decisions in the midst of a crisis.

The provision of accurate knowledge is an important determinant in whether panic will occur. Even if the news is very bad, knowledge is preferable to uncertainty in which fantasies and rumors run rampant. Providing inaccurate news or lying to the public results in loss of credibility that cannot be regained, as was seen at Three Mile Island and in Surat, India.

Untrained or mistrained responders can cause group breakdown and institutional panic, which would not be reassuring to the public if it occurred in a hospital, for example. There are several factors that could contribute to group disorganization and institutional breakdown:

- distrust prior to the event,
- a breakdown in communication,
- failure of critical elements,
- poor leadership, and
- a perception that there is no effective response.

Realistic simulation training maximizes the probability of people performing their roles well by identifying key personnel and facilitating the development of personal relationships. It minimizes panic by teaching decision-making and problem-solving skills under calm conditions, rather than during the chaotic time of an actual response.

While panic may not be evident during a crisis, there will likely be significant numbers of the "worried well" seeking medical evaluation. The signs and symptoms of anxiety are protean and ubiquitous. People who have been exposed to infection often worry that they are becoming ill when they experience anxiety symptoms. Following an outbreak, well-designed risk communication can reassure low-risk citizens that they are not sick, thereby reducing the number of people seeking hospital evaluation.

Now, despite having devoted so much time to a discussion of the multidimensional nature of panic, it may be wise to strike the word "panic" from our lexicons. Telling people not to panic may, in fact, reinforce the behaviors we are trying to prevent. Also, in terms of trying to understand and develop predictive models about how the public will behave, it is far more helpful to explicitly describe the behaviors rather than lumping them under the rubric of "panic."

Historical Examples and Post-Outbreak Interventions

Following the SCUD attacks on Israel during the Gulf War, for every ill or injured casualty seeking medical assistance, there were four non-ill behavioral casualties seeking aid. This phenomenon has also been observed during disease outbreaks. Furthermore, medical and hospital support personnel are not immune from fear-organized behaviors, such as absenteeism and decreased performance, especially in circumstances where emergency and health personnel are worried about their families.

The 1994 outbreak of pneumonic plague in Surat, India, illustrates how fear-organized behaviors can dominate the public's response to an epidemic. This is true despite the fact that, in this case, the organism was susceptible to antibiotics. Stigma and social isolation had economic as well as psychological consequences, and fear of disease dissemination eroded feelings of safety in many parts of the world. Communicating the risks and managing fear, anger, and paranoia should be major intervention objectives in the wake of a post-eradication outbreak.

Overdedication—people continuing to work despite suffering the effects of fatigue from sleep deprivation and intense mental and physical activity—is a common problem in crisis situations. There are scores of case examples in which exhausted leaders have made poor decisions which have endangered others. Protocols need to specify plans for rotating all personnel. This is especially critical in situations in which the outbreak may extend from days to weeks to months.

The tendency of the science community to debate and criticize as a way of seeking the truth will not reassure the public and may actually lead to the loss of credibility. A number of experts have emphasized the need for "one voice" to provide information to the public. While this is a laudable goal, it may be unreachable given the long-standing traditions of scientific discourse. We need a better understanding of how the public should be trained to anticipate and cope with the diverse, and often conflicting, information that will be disseminated in the wake of an outbreak. For example, following the midwestern U.S. floods in 1997, there were discrepancies in the amount of time residents were told to boil their water by different government agencies. In the face of this confusion, how did people decide what to do? Discrepancies between what leaders and experts are telling people to do and what they, themselves, are doing, will not escape media notice and will undermine the credibility of the authorities.

Recommendations

- Multiple research methodologies must be employed to address the psychological and behavioral consequences of a post-eradication outbreak.
- Policies on the distribution of limited resources, such as vaccine and antibiotics, should be informed by behavioral research and ethical review.
- Planning for the behavioral and psychosocial aftermath of a post-eradication outbreak requires a multidisciplinary effort involving political, medical and mental health leaders, governmental and social institutions, and the citizenry.
- While developing outbreak policies, the emotional and physical impact of a major disease outbreak on leaders must be taken into account in order to ensure rational, informed decision-making during the crisis.
- Research should be directed toward delineating how best to enlist media support in the management of outbreaks.
- The behavioral and societal effects of past infectious disease outbreaks should be studied systematically and a taxonomy developed which can be used to identify the effects and course of responses to outbreaks. These studies should examine responses in individuals, families, small groups, hospitals, and communities. The review should also examine the response to past uses of mass quarantine, evacuation, immunization, and isolation. Information gleaned from these studies can serve as the basis for hypotheses which can be tested in future outbreaks.
- Infectious disease specialists, risk communication experts, public officials, and members of the media should develop communication and information programs for each disease of concern. Effective risk communication after an attack will be key in promoting healthy and constructive public behaviors and reducing fear-organized behaviors. These programs should designate who will inform the public, and they should delineate the specific actions recommended for citizens to minimize their possibility of falling ill. Messages must be specifically designed for each segment of the population, based on available information and input from credible community leaders.

POST-ERADICATION CHALLENGES IN THE DEVELOPING WORLD

Ellyn W. Ogden, M.P.H.

Worldwide Polio Eradication Coordinator and Senior Technical Advisor for Health and Child Survival, Bureau for Global Programs U.S. Agency for International Development, Washington, D.C.

The U.S. Agency for International Development (USAID) provides foreign assistance to developing countries and maintains offices and ongoing programs in nearly every country of the developing world. Immunization has long been a hallmark of AID's child survival activities. In 1996, at the urging of Rotary International, Congress directed USAID to establish a global polio eradication program that would provide a minimum of $25 million per year for polio-specific activities. The rationale for this earmark was based on the success of the eradication efforts in the Americas, where USAID had been the largest external donor, and on the belief that savings would come once vaccination could stop. Annual estimated savings from vaccination costs alone ranged from $230 million per year in the United States to $1.5 billion globally, in perpetuity, once immunization ceased. Because of a complex budget structure and earmarks for USAID, much of the funding had to come out of existing resources, primarily routine immunization programs. Knowing the enormous challenge of immunizing children and establishing certification-standard surveillance in the most difficult-to-reach areas of Africa and South Asia, often under conflict situations, as well as concerns regarding cessation of immunization, USAID entered into this commitment with skepticism. However, once engaged, the commitment has been strong and visible, with hopes that USAID, working closely with its partner organizations, would leave a long-term legacy behind.

I have listened carefully to the presentations over the last few days and the doubts being raised about the feasibility of stopping polio immunization. If true, USAID is in a very difficult position. We have pledged to maintain political, financial, and technical involvement until the world is certified polio-free, even if the road is bumpier and longer than originally planned. Any lessening of the effort at this point in the eradication program would be a signal to other donors and to host country governments that they can retreat. This risks halting the momentum currently enjoyed by the program as well as setting the stage for polio cases to resurge to pre-eradication levels—100 times what they are today. USAID does not want to send this signal without seriously considering all of the scientific data and opinions, how the public and Congress would perceive it, and what it would mean in terms of USAID's credibility.

While many reputable scientists and virologists are firm in their belief that polio eradication is feasible and immunization can safely stop at some point in the near future, others, equally strongly, believe that polio immunization may never cease. If the funds spent on eradication cannot be recouped, then how do we tell our constituents—the children in developing countries—that we have invested nearly $1.8 billion thus far, and that this amount is increasing, for an activity that may never be stopped. In the meantime, in a district in Zambia, for example, it costs about $11 per capita to provide an essential package of basic health services, but currently available resources amount to only $5 per capita. Access by developing countries to limited supplies of vaccine stockpiles and costs to contain potential outbreaks in the post-eradication era, raise additional issues of equity and public health priority.

This is a very serious issue. The need for eradication and anticipating post-eradication needs must be balanced with the general health needs of the children, while at the same time maintaining USAID's integrity and credibility in the eyes of the public, Congress, host countries, and other stakeholders.

There are a number of other important issues that must also be addressed while considering eradication. Eradication programs have consequences, both opportunities and threats, beyond wiping out a virus. First, the great need to provide every child with basic preventive health care, including immunization. House-to-house strategies are no longer enough for delivering polio vaccine, so USAID and its partners are now going child-to-child, which requires intensive effort looking for children in places where we have never looked before. Like the homeless here on the streets in Washington, D.C., it is easy to simply walk by them. But we cannot do this in the slums of Calcutta, for example. To achieve polio eradication we must find and immunize every child. Once we find them how can we ignore them for other services? How do we bring the same intensity of effort and find the resources to bring basic preventive services to them as well?

Second, polio eradication is helping to build or revitalize many aspects of health infrastructure in developing countries. One example is the important area of communications. Most laboratories in developing countries did not have dedicated phone and fax lines until USAID helped pay for them in their effort to establish an effective laboratory network for acute flaccid paralysis (AFP) surveillance. With foresight and planning, the laboratory network will extend beyond AFP, but in order for this to happen, objectives need to be outlined from the beginning. Even if eradication efforts fail, the network is a legacy that must continue if we are ever to build a stronger system of health services. It is this type of global communication system that will alert us to outbreaks of disease and enable us to take corrective action. USAID considers this a good investment for polio eradication and for protecting the United States.

Finally, conflict situations are posing tremendous challenges in many developing countries. In the Eastern Congo, for example, administering vaccinations requires negotiating with the Congolese rebels to set aside certain days of peace—something I have personally done. Despite all good-faith negotiations, it is impossible to control all factions or undisciplined soldiers who shoot anybody they see. Everyone from volunteers, to health workers, to staff of U.N. organizations, to donors, regularly demonstrate acts of courage and put themselves at risk in an effort to vaccinate children. Sometimes, these acts of bravery are a step toward peace-building. Sometimes, vaccinators die while conducting eradication activities. CDC, to their credit, has established a Heroes Fund for the many vaccinators who have died since polio eradication started. We should not enter eradication efforts lightly without thinking of these people who are giving up their lives for the sake of eradication.

USAID is proud of our involvement in polio eradication and our contribution to reducing the death, disability, and social stigma that accompanies the disease. The global program can be proud of the success so far; thousands of cases of polio have been prevented; children that might have been paralyzed are walking, will marry, be involved in economic activities, and be vital members of their communities. USAID leadership to maximize the benefits of polio eradication, to raise awareness of the health needs of children, and to seek peace will have provided a great service—regardless of whether immunization can cease or not.

REFERENCES

Alibek K. 1999. *Biohazard.* New York: Random House.

Bentley J. 2000. Hospital Preparedness, Presentation at the Second National Symposium on Medical and Public Health Response to Bioterrorism, Washington, D.C., November 28–29, 2000.

Centers for Disease Control and Prevention. 1992. Public sector vaccination efforts in response to the resurgence of measles among preschool-age children—United States—1989–1991. *Morbidity and Mortality Weekly Report* 41(29):522–525.

Fidler D. 2000. Legal Issues Surrounding Public Health Emergencies, Presentation at the Second National Symposium on Medical and Public Health Response to Bioterrorism, Washington, D.C., November 28–29, 2000.

Garrett L. 1994. Pp. 175–176 in The Coming Plague: Newly Emerging Diseases in a World Out of Balance. New York: Penguin Books.

Gremillion DH and Crawford GE. 1981. Measles pneumonia in young adults: An analysis of 106 cases. *American Journal of Medicine* 71:539–542.

Henderson DA, Inglesby TV, Bartlett JG, Ascher MS, Eitzen E, Jahrling PB, Hauer J, Layton M, McDade J, Osterholm MT, O'Toole T, Parker G, Perl T, Russell PK, and Tonat K. 1999. Smallpox as a biological weapon: medical and public health management. *Journal of the American Medical Association* 281:2127–2137.

Inglesby T, Grossman R, and O'Toole T. 2001. A plague on your city: Observations from TOPOFF. *Clinical Infectious Diseases* 32(3):436–445.

LeDuc JW and Becher J. 1999. Current status of smallpox vaccine. *Emerging Infectious Diseases* 5:593–594.

Markowitz LE and Katz SL. 1994. Measles vaccine In Plotkin, SA and Mortimer, EA, (eds.) *Vaccines*, p. 248. Philadelphia: WB Saunders.

Osterholm MT and Schwartz J. 2000. *Living Terrors*. New York: Delacourte Press.

O'Toole T. 2000. Biological Weapons: National Security Threat and Public Health Emergency, CSIS Presentation, Washington, D.C., August 22, 2000, p. 10.

Appendix A

Glossary and Acronyms

GLOSSARY

This glossary is intended to define terms commonly encountered throughout this report as well as some terms that are commonly used in the public health arena. This glossary is not all inclusive. New terms and new usages of existing terms will emerge with time and with advances in technology. The definitions for the terms presented here were compiled from a multitude of sources.

Adenovirus: A group of viruses responsible for a spectrum of respiratory disease as well as infection of the stomach and intestine, eyes, and bladder. Patients with compromised immune systems are especially susceptible to severe complications of adenovirus infection. Adenoviruses are transmitted by direct contact, fecal-oral transmission, and occasionally waterborne transmission. Shedding of the virus can occur for months or years after the initial infection.

Anthropogenic: Of, relating to, or resulting from the influence of human beings on nature.

Antibiotic: Class of substances or chemicals that can kill or inhibit the growth of bacteria. Originally antibiotics were derived from natural sources (e.g., penicillin was derived from molds), but many currently used antibiotics are semisynthetic and are modified by the addition of artificial chemical components.

Antibiotic resistance: Property of bacteria that confers the capacity to inactivate or exclude antibiotics or a mechanism that blocks the inhibitory or killing effects of antibiotics.

Antimicrobial agents: Class of substances that can destroy or inhibit the growth of pathogenic groups of microorganisms, including bacteria, viruses, parasites, and fungi.

Apoptosis: A genetically determined process of intracellular cell destruction postulated to exist and to be activated by a stimulus or by the removal of a suppressing agent or stimulus in order to explain the orderly breakdown and elimination of superfluous or unwanted cells (as immune cells targeted against the self in the development of self-tolerance or larval cells in amphibians undergoing metamorphosis)—also called *programmed cell death.*

Arenaviruses: Any of a group of viruses containing a single strand of RNA, having a grainy appearance due to the presence of ribosomes in the virion, and including the Machupo virus and the causative agents of lymphocytic choriomeningitis and Lassa fever.

Attenuate: To reduce the severity of (a disease) or virulence or vitality of (a pathogenic agent).

Bacteremia: The presence of bacteria in the bloodstream.

Bacteria: Microscopic, single-celled organisms that have some biochemical and structural features different from those of animal and plant cells.

Bacteriophage: A virus that infects bacteria—called also phage.

Basic research: Fundamental, theoretical, or experimental investigation to advance scientific knowledge, with immediate practical application not being a direct objective.

Benchmark: For a particular indicator or performance goal, the industry measure of best performance. The benchmarking process identifies the best performance in the industry (health care or non-health care) for a particular process or outcome, determines how that performance is achieved, and applies the lessons learned to improve performance.

Broad-spectrum antibiotic: An antibiotic effective against a large number of bacterial species. It generally describes antibiotics effective against both gram-positive and gram-negative classes of bacteria.

BSL (biosafety level): Specific combinations of work practices, safety equipment, and facilities, designed to minimize the exposure of workers and the environment to infectious agents. Biosafety level 1 applies to agents that do not ordinarily cause human disease. Biosafety level 2 is appropriate for agents that can cause human disease, but whose potential for transmission is limited. Biosafety level 3 applies to agents that may be transmitted by the respiratory route which can cause serious infection. Biosafety level 4 is used for the diagnosis of exotic agents that pose a high risk of life-threatening disease, which may be transmitted by the aerosol route and for which there is no vaccine or therapy.

BT (bioterrorism): Terrorism using biologic agents. Biological diseases and the agents that might be used for terrorism have been listed by the CDC and comprise viruses, bacteria, rickettsiae, fungi and biological toxins. These agents have been classified according to the degree of danger each agent is felt to pose into one of three categories: A, B, and C.

CDC (Centers for Disease Control and Prevention): A public health agency of the U.S. Department of Health and Human Services whose mission is to promote health and quality of life by preventing and controlling disease, injury, and disability.

Clinical practice guidelines: Systematically developed statements that assist practitioners and patients with decision making about appropriate health care for specific clinical circumstances.

Clinical research: Investigations aimed at translating basic, fundamental science into medical practice.

Clinical trials: As used in this report, research with human volunteers to establish the safety and efficacy of a drug, such as an antibiotic or a vaccine.

Clinician: One qualified or engaged in the clinical practice of medicine, psychiatry, or psychology, as distinguished from one specializing in laboratory or research techniques in the same fields.

Coxsackievirus: Any of several enteroviruses associated with human diseases (as meningitis or herpangina).

CRS (congenital rubella syndrome): The constellation of abnormalities caused by infection with the rubella (German measles) virus before birth. The syndrome is characterized by multiple congenital malformations (birth defects) and mental retardation.

Cytokine: A small protein released by cells that has a specific effect on the interactions between cells, on communications between cells or on the behavior of cells. The cytokines include the interleukins, lymphokines and cell signal molecules, such as tumor necrosis factor and the interferons, which trigger inflammation and respond to infections.

DHHS (U.S. Department of Health and Human Services): The U.S. government's principal agency for protecting the health of all Americans and providing essential human services, especially for those who are least able to help themselves (www.os.dhhs.gov).

DoD (U.S. Department of Defense): DoD trains and equips the armed forces through three military departments—the Army, Navy, and Air Force whose primary job is to train and equip their personnel to perform warfighting, peacekeeping and humanitarian/disaster assistance tasks.

Echovirus: One of a group of viruses found in the gastrointestinal tract. The "echo" part of the name stands for enteric cytopathic human orphan viruses. "Orphan" implied that they were viruses not associated with any disease. Now, however, it is known that echoviruses can cause meningitis, intestinal infection, pericarditis (inflammation of the membrane around the heart) and upper respiratory infections.

ELISA (enzyme-linked immunosorbent assay): A rapid immunochemical test utilized to detect substances that have antigenic properties, primarily proteins. ELISA tests are generally highly sensitive and specific.

Emerging infections: Any infectious disease that has come to medical attention within the last two decades or for which there is a threat that its prevalence will increase in the near future. Many times, such diseases exist in nature as zoonoses and emerge as human pathogens only when humans come into contact with a formerly isolated animal population, such as monkeys in a rain forest that are no longer isolated because of deforestation. Drug-resistant organisms could also be included as the cause of emerging infections since they exist because of human influence. Some recent examples of agents responsible for emerging infections include human immunodeficiency virus, Ebola virus, and multidrug-resistant *Mycobacterium tuberculosis.*

Encephalitis: An acute inflammatory disease of the brain due to direct viral invasion or to hypersensitivity initiated by a virus or other foreign protein.

Endemic: Disease that is present in a community or common among a group of people; said of a disease continually prevailing in a region.

Enterovirus: A virus that comes into the body through the gastrointestinal tract and thrives there, often moving on to attack the nervous system. Enteroviruses include the polioviruses, rhinoviruses, and echoviruses.

Enzootic: A disease of low morbidity that is constantly present in an animal community.

Epizootic: A disease of high morbidity that is only occasionally present in an animal community.

Etiology: Science and study of the causes of diseases and their mode of operation.

FDA (U.S. Food and Drug Administration): A public health agency of the U.S. Department of Health and Human Services charged with protecting American consumers by enforcing the Federal Food, Drug, and Cosmetic Act and several related health laws.

Flavivirus: Any of a group of arboviruses that contain a single strand of RNA, are transmitted by ticks and mosquitoes, and include the causative agents of dengue, Japanese B encephalitis, and yellow fever.

Hantavirus: A group of viruses that cause hemorrhagic fever and pneumonia. Hantaviruses are transmitted to humans by contact direct or indirectly with the saliva and excreta of rodents such as deer mice, field mice, and ground voles.

Hepatosplenomegaly: Coincident enlargement of the liver and spleen.

Herd immunity: A reduction in the probability of infection that is held to apply to susceptible members of a population in which a significant proportion of the individuals are immune because the chance of coming in contact with an infected individual is less.

IFN (interferon): A naturally occurring substance that interferes with the ability of viruses to reproduce. Interferon also boosts the immune system. There are a number of different interferons and they fall into three main classes: alpha, beta, and gamma. All are proteins (lymphokines) normally produced by the body in response to infection. The interferons have been synthesized using recombinant DNA technology.

IgG: A class of antibodies including those most commonly circulating in the blood and active especially against bacteria, viruses, and proteins foreign to the body—also called *immunoglobulin G*.

IgM: A class of antibodies of high molecular weight including those that appear early in the immune response to be replaced later by IgG of lower molecular weight, are capable of binding complement, and do not cross the placenta—also called *immunoglobulin M*.

Immunogenicity: The property that endows a substance with the capacity to provoke an immune response or the degree to which a substance possesses this property.

Incidence: The frequency of new occurrences of disease within a defined time interval. Incidence rate is the number of new cases of a specified disease divided by the number of people in a population over a specified period of time, usually 1 year.

Infection: The invasion of the body or a part of the body by a pathogenic agent, such as a microoganism or virus. Under favorable conditions the agent develops or multiplies, the results of which may produce injurious effects. Infection should not be confused with disease.

IPV (inactivated polio vaccine): A vaccine for polio given as a shot in the arm or leg. The polio virus in IPV has been inactivated (killed). Also called the Salk vaccine.

Lentivirus: Any of a group of retroviruses that cause slowly progressive often fatal animal diseases (as AIDS).

Macrophages: A type of white blood cell that ingests foreign material. Macrophages are key players in the immune response to foreign invaders such as infectious microorganisms.

Meningoencephalitis: Inflammation of the brain and meninges—also called *encephalomeningitis.*

MHC (major histocompatibility complex): A cluster of genes on chromosome 6 concerned with antigen production and critical to transplantation.

Microcephaly: A condition of abnormal smallness of the head usually associated with mental retardation.

Monoclonal antibodies: Identical antibodies that are made in large amounts in the laboratory. Doctors are studying ways of using monoclonal antibodies to treat leukemia.

NCID (National Center for Infectious Diseases): Its mission is to prevent illness, disability, and death caused by infectious diseases in the US and around the world. NCID conducts surveillance, epidemic investigations, epidemiological and laboratory research, training, and public education programs to develop, evaluate, and promote prevention and control strategies for infectious diseases.

Neurovirulence: The tendency or capacity of a microorganism to cause disease of the nervous system.

NIAID (National Institute of Allergy and Infectious Diseases): A division of NIH that provides the major support for scientists conducting research aimed at developing better ways to diagnose, treat, and prevent the many infectious, immunological, and allergenic diseases that afflict people worldwide.

NIH (National Institutes of Health): A public health agency of the U.S. Department of Health and Human Services whose goal is to acquire new knowledge to help prevent, detect, diagnose, and treat disease and disability, from the rarest genetic disorder to the common cold.

NK (natural killer) cell: A large granular lymphocyte capable of killing a tumor or microbial cell without prior exposure to the target cell and without having it presented with or marked by a histocompatibility antigen.

OPV (oral polio vaccine): A vaccine for polio, given by mouth, and preferred for most children.

PAHO (Pan American Health Organization): An international public health agency with almost 100 years of experience working to improve health and living standards of the people of the Americas. It enjoys international recognition as part of the United Nations system, serving as the

Regional Office for the Americas of the World Health Organization, and as the health organization of the Inter-American System.

Pandemic: Occurring over a wide geographic area and affecting an exceptionally high proportion of the population.

Parvoviruses: A group of extremely small, morphologically similar, ether-resistant, DNA viruses; the group includes the osteolytic hamster viruses and adeno-associated viruses.

PDA (patent ductus arteriosus): An abnormal condition in which the ductus arteriosus fails to close after birth.

Prions: A newly discovered type of disease-causing agent, neither bacterial nor fungal nor viral, and containing no genetic material. A prion is a protein that occurs normally in a harmless form. By folding into an aberrant shape, the normal prion turns into a rogue agent. It then coopts other normal prions to become rogue prions.They have been held responsible for a number of degenerative brain diseases, including mad cow disease, Creutzfeldt-Jacob disease, and possibly some cases of Alzheimer's disease.

Prophylactic antibiotics: Antibiotics that are administered before evidence of infection with the intention of warding off disease.

Purpura: Any of several hemorrhagic states characterized by patches of purplish discoloration resulting from extravasation of blood into the skin and mucous membranes.

Radiolucent: Partly or wholly permeable to radiation and especially X rays.

RSV (respiratory syncytial virus): A virus that causes mild respiratory infections in adults but in young children can produce severe respiratory problems. Effective immunity against RSV requires a continuous solid level of antibodies against the virus.

Seroconversion: The production of antibodies in response to an antigen.

Seronegative: Having or being a negative serum reaction especially in a test for the presence of an antibody.

Seropositive: Having or being a positive serum reaction especially in a test for the presence of an antibody.

Seroprevalence: The frequency of individuals in a population that have a particular element (as antibodies to HIV) in their blood serum.

Serotype: The kind of microorganism as characterized by serologic typing (testing for recognizable antigens on the surface of the microorganism).

Surveillance systems: Used in this report to refer to data collection and recordkeeping to track the emergence and spread of disease-causing organisms such as antibiotic-resistant bacteria.

TOPOFF: An exercise conducted by the Department of Justice which engaged key personnel in the management of mock chemical, biological, or cyberterrorist attacks. So named because it involved the participation of top officials of the U.S. government.

USAID (U.S. Agency for International Development): An independent federal government agency that receives overall foreign policy guidance from the Secretary of State. The agency works to support long-term, equitable economic growth and to advance U.S. foreign policy objectives by supporting global health, democracy, conflict prevention, and humanitarian assistance initiatives.

USAMRIID (U.S. Army Medical Research Institute of Infectious Diseases): It is the lead medical research laboratory for the U.S. Biological Defense Research Program which conducts research to develop strategies, products, information, procedures, and training programs for medical defense against biological warfare threats and naturally occurring infectious diseases that require special containment. It is an organization of the U.S. Army Medical Research and Materiel Command (USAMRMC).

USDA (U.S. Department of Agriculture): Founded in 1862, its mission is to enhance the quality of life for the American people by supporting production of agriculture and ensuring a safe, affordable, nutritious, and accessible food supply.

VA (Department of Veterans Affairs): A cabinet-level department that has the care of veterans as its primary mission and is composed of 3 administrations: Veterans Health Administration, Veterans Benefit Administration, and National Cemetery Administration.

Vaccine: A preparation of living, attenuated, or killed bacteria or viruses, fractions thereof, or synthesized or recombinant antigens identical or similar to those found in the disease-causing organisms that is administered to raise immunity to a particular microorganism.

VHF (viral hemorrhagic fevers): A group of illnesses that are caused by viruses of four distinct families: arenaviruses, filoviruses, bunyaviruses, and flaviviruses.

Viremia: The presence of virus in the blood of a host.

Virulence: The ability of any infectious agent to produce disease. The virulence of a microoganism (such as a bacterium or virus) is a measure of the severity of the disease it is capable of causing.

WHO (World Health Organization): Its objective is the attainment by all peoples of the highest possible level of health, a state of complete physical, mental, and social well-being and not merely the absence of disease or infirmity. WHO also proposes conventions, agreements, regulations, and makes recommendations about international nomenclature of diseases, causes of death and public health practices. It develops, establishes, and promotes international standards concerning foods and biological, pharmaceutical, and similar substances.

Xenogeneic: Derived from, originating in, or being a member of another species.

Zoonotic disease or infection: An infection or infectious disease that may be transmitted from vertebrate animals (e.g., a rodent) to humans.

ACRONYMS

AFP	acute flaccid paralysis
BRC	Biological Resource Centers
BWTC	Biological Weapons and Toxins Convention
DMORT	Disaster Mortuary Operational Response Team
DPT	diptheria-pertussis-tetanus
EMTALA	Emergency Medical Treatment and Labor Act
EPI	Expanded Programme on Immunization
GAVI	Global Alliance for Vaccines and Immunization
GIDs	global immunization days
IHR	International Health Regulations
JCAHO	Joint Commission on the Accreditation of Health Care Organizations
JIC	Joint Information Center
JOC	Joint Operations Center
MMR	measles-mumps-rubella
NIDs	national immunization days
PCR	polymerase chain reaction
SIV	simian immunodeficiency virus
TNF	tumor necrosis factor

VAPP	vaccine-associated paralytic poliovirus
WER	*Weekly Epidemiological Record*
WHA	World Health Assembly

APPENDIX B
Workshop Agenda The Consequences of Viral Disease Eradication: Addressing Post-Immunization Challenges

February 1–2, 2001
Lecture Room
National Academy of Sciences
2101 Constitution Avenue, N.W., Washington, DC

Thursday, February 1, 2001

8:30 Continental Breakfast

9:00 **Welcome and workshop introduction**
Joshua Lederberg, Ph.D.
Chair, Forum on Emerging Infections
Sackler Foundation Scholar and Nobel Laureate
The Rockefeller University, New York, NY

9:15 **Keynote address**
History and Prospects for Disease Eradication
Ciro de Quadros, M.D., M.P.H.
Director, Division of Vaccines and Immunization
Pan American Health Organization, Washington, DC

Session I: Case Studies of Major Eradication or Elimination Efforts

This session will address the standards and strategies, technical feasibility, political will, and financial commitment for several diseases targeted for eradication or elimination. Discussions will identify the successes and failures of these efforts, and the challenges for post-eradication/elimination strategies.

10:00 **Smallpox**
Donald A. Henderson, M.D., M.P.H.
Director, Center for Civilian Biodefense Studies
The Johns Hopkins University, Baltimore, MD

10:30 **Break**

10:45 **The next target after polio: Global eradication of measles**
Stephen Cochi, M.D., M.P.H.
Director, Vaccine-Preventable Disease Eradication Division
National Immunization Program, Centers for Disease Control and Prevention, Atlanta GA

11:15 **Eradication of congenital rubella syndrome**
Stanley A. Plotkin, M.D.
Aventis Pasteur, Swiftwater, PA

11:45 **Post-polio eradication: Issues and challenges**
Walter R. Dowdle, M.D.
Public Health Consultant
Task Force for Child Survival and Development, Atlanta, GA

12:15 **Lunch**

Session II: Biologic Challenges to Post-Eradication

This session will address the science-based underpinnings of how and when to stop immunization, and the protective actions that remain to be established. We will examine the current state-of-the-science of several diseases poised for elimination/eradication and identify gaps in our knowledge, primarily focusing on the risk of pathogen transmission to and maintenance in susceptible individuals. Through the issues discussed we will identify the effect they have on the duration of disease elimination/eradication programs, as well as the likelihood for their success.

1:30 **Duration of infection, recrudescence, and environmental stability of pathogens targeted for elimination**
Professor Roy Anderson
Chair, Department of Infectious Disease Epidemiology
Imperial College School of Medicine, London, UK

2:15 **Laboratory specimens, genetic research, bio-engineering, and the danger of malice**
C.J. Peters, M.D.
Professor, Departments of Pathology, and Microbiology and Immunology
Center for Tropical Diseases, University of Texas Medical Branch, Galveston, TX

2.45 **Break**

3:00 **Natural SIV reservoirs and human zoonotic risk**
Beatrice H. Hahn, M.D.
Professor, Departments of Medicine and Microbiology
University of Alabama, Birmingham, AL

3:30 **Vaccine-associated cases**
Jeffrey I. Cohen, M.D
Head, Medical Virology Section, Laboratory of Clinical Investigation
National Institute of Allergy and Infectious Diseases, National Institutes of Health, Bethesda, MD

4:00 **Adjourn public session**

Friday, February 2, 2001

7:30 Continental Breakfast

8:00 **Opening remarks**
Joshua Lederberg, Ph.D.
Chair, Forum on Emerging Infections

Session III: Challenges to Post-Eradication Operational and Institutional Remediation

The need for resources will likely increase for countries with multiple eradication campaigns, particularly as disease prevalence decreases and surveillance intensifies. This session will address the thoroughness with which public health systems and laboratories are able to define their limitations and manage their resources.

8:15 **International health regulations and quarantine**
Marlo Libel, M.D.
Division of Disease Prevention and Control
Pan American Health Organization, Washington, DC

9:00 **Disease surveillance, program management, and sustainability of immunization programs**
Donald S. Burke, M.D.
Professor and Director, Center for Immunization Research, Department of International Health
School of Hygiene and Public Health, The Johns Hopkins University, Baltimore, MD

9:30 **The capacity of public health services to respond to an outbreak in the post-eradication era**
Carl E. Taylor, M.D., M.P.H.
Professor Emeritus, Department of International Health
School of Hygiene and Public Health, The Johns Hopkins University, Baltimore, MD

10:00 **Laboratory security and regulations governing viral pathogenesis in a post-immunization era**
Raymond H. Cypess, D.V.M., Ph.D.
President and CEO
American Type Culture Collection (ATCC), Manassas, VA
Frank Simione, M.S.
American Type Culture Collection (ATCC), Manassas, VA

10:30 **Break**

Session IV: Medical Intervention and Technological Solutions

Many of the vaccines and drugs available today are the same ones that have been used for decades. This session will review the present vaccine and drug armamentaria with a view toward improving their safety, efficacy and potential value against diseases targeted for eradication.

10:45 **The polio eradication effort: should vaccine eradication be next?**
Vincent R. Racaniello, Ph.D.
Higgins Professor, Department of Microbiology, and Editor, Journal of Virology
Columbia University College of Physicians & Surgeons, New York, NY

11:15 **Antiviral therapy in the management of post-eradication outbreaks**
Richard J. Whitley, M.D.
Professor, Department of Pediatrics
Ambulatory Care Center, School of Medicine, University of Alabama, South Birmingham, AL

11:45 **Passive antibody and immune-enhancement strategies**
Diane E. Griffin, M.D., Ph.D.
Professor and Chair, Department of Molecular Microbiology and Immunology
School of Hygiene and Public Health, The Johns Hopkins University, Baltimore, MD

12:15 **The potential role of probiotics and microbial ecology in host defense**
Susanna Cunningham-Rundles, Ph.D.
Professor of Immunology
Weill Medical College of Cornell University, New York, NY

12:45 **Lunch**

Session V: The Response to Post-Eradication Outbreaks

Protecting populations that are no longer immune presents formidable challenges to public health agencies, pharmaceutical manufacturers, security analysts, and the public. Resolution of these issues in advance affects when and how prevention activities can be stopped in conjunction with disease eradication.

1:30 **Preparedness of the U.S. health care system to respond to disease outbreaks**
Ken Bloem, M.D.
Senior Fellow, The Johns Hopkins Center for Civilian Biodefense Studies
Former CEO, Georgetown Medical Center

2:00 **Vaccines for post-elimination (eradication) contingencies**
Thomas Monath, M.D.
Vice President, Research and Medical Affairs
Acambis Inc. (formerly OraVax, Inc.), Cambridge, MA

2:30 **Strategic priorities for addressing post-eradication outbreaks**
Robert Kadlec, M.D., M.T.M.H.
Colonel, US Air Force, and Professor, Military Strategy and Operations
National War College, National Defense University, Washington, D.C.

3:00 **Understanding the public and media response to an outbreak**
Ann E. Norwood, M.D.
Colonel, US Army, Associate Professor and Associate Chair
Department of Psychiatry, Uniformed Services University of the Health Sciences, Bethesda, MD

3:30 **The post-eradication research agenda**
Joshua Lederberg, Ph.D.
Chair, Forum on Emerging Infections
Sackler Foundation Scholar, and Nobel Laureate
The Rockefeller University, New York, NY

4:00 **Break**

Session VI:
Panel Session: Identifying the Threats and Mitigating the Impact

The challenges and opportunities facing disease eradication and how they will affect public policy will be identified through an open discussion among invited panelists, Forum members, speakers, and the workshop audience. Issues to address will include the identification of possible requirements that need to be met prior to eradication, such as collections of diverse isolates and strains, an organism's complete genomic sequence, full understanding of the life history of the organism and its mechanism(s) of pathogenesis, legal issues and authorities surrounding the response to an epidemic; and the ethical considerations pertaining to cessation of immunization, as well as preserving biodiversity versus species extinction.

Co-Moderators:

Joshua Lederberg, Ph.D. Chair, Forum on Emerging Infections
Margaret Hamburg, M.D., Assistant Secretary for Planning and Evaluation, U.S. Department of Health and Human Services

Invited Panelists:

Gail Cassell, Vice President, Infectious Diseases, Drug Discovery Research and Clinical Investigation, Eli Lilly & Company, Indianapolis, IN
Michael Osterholm, Chairman and CEO, Infection Control Advisory Network, Inc., Eden Prairie, MN
Stephen Teret J.D, Professor, Program on Law and Public Health, The Johns Hopkins School of Hygiene and Public Health, Baltimore, MD
Samuel L. Katz, M.D., D.Sc., Chairman of the Board, Burroughs Wellcome Fund, and; Wilburt C. Davison Professor & Chairman Emeritus, Department of Pediatrics, Duke University Medical Center, Durham, NC
Ellyn W. Ogden, MPH, Worldwide Polio Eradication Coordinator and Senior Technical Advisor in Health and Child Survival, Bureau for Global Programs, U.S. Agency for International Development, Washington, D.C.

4:15 **Panel discussion, perspectives from different communities, and synthesis**

5:30 **Closing remarks**
Joshua Lederberg, Ph.D.
Chair, Forum on Emerging Infections
Sackler Foundation Scholar, and Nobel Laureate
The Rockefeller University, New York, NY

5:45 **Adjournment**

APPENDIX

C

Forum Member and Speaker Biographies

FORUM MEMBERS

JOSHUA LEDERBERG, Ph.D. (*Chair*), is professor emeritus of molecular genetics and informatics and Sackler Foundation Scholar at the Rockefeller University, New York, NY. His lifelong research, for which he received the Nobel Prize in 1958, has been in genetic structure and function in microorganisms. He has a keen interest in international health and was cochair of a previous Institute of Medicine Committee on Emerging Microbial Threats to Health (1990–1992) and currently is cochair of the Committee on Emerging Microbial Threats to Health in the 21st Century. He has been a member of the National Academy of Sciences since 1957 and is a charter member of the Institute of Medicine.

STEVEN J. BRICKNER, Ph.D., is research advisor for antibacterials chemistry at Pfizer Global Research and Development. He received his Ph.D. in organic chemistry from Cornell University and was an NIH postdoctoral research fellow at the University of Wisconsin-Madison. Dr. Brickner is a medicinal chemist with nearly 20 years of research experience in the pharmaceutical industry, all focused on the discovery and development of novel antibacterial agents. He is an inventor/coinventor on 21 U.S. patents and has published numerous scientific papers, primarily in the area of the oxazolidinones. Prior to joining Pfizer in 1996, he led a team at Pharmacia and Upjohn that discovered and developed linezolid, the first member of a new class of antibiotics to be approved in the last 35 years.

GAIL H. CASSELL, Ph.D., is vice president of infectious diseases research, drug discovery research, and clinical investigation at Eli Lilly & Company. Previously, she was the Charles H. McCauley professor and (since 1987) chair of the Department of Microbiology, University of Alabama, Schools of Medicine and Dentistry, Birmingham, a department which, under her leadership, has ranked first in research funding from the National Institutes of Health since 1989. She is a member of the Director's Advisory Committee of the Centers for Disease Control and Prevention. Dr. Cassell is past president of the American Society for Microbiology (ASM) and is serving her third three-year term as chairman of the Public and Scientific Affairs Board of ASM. She is a former member of the National Institutes of Health Director's Advisory Committee and a former member of the Advisory Council of the National Institute of Allergy and Infectious Diseases. She has also served as an adviser on infectious diseases and indirect costs of research to the White House Office on Science and Technology and was previously chair of the Board of Scientific Counselors of the National Center for Infectious Diseases, Centers for Disease Control and Prevention. Dr. Cassell served eight years on the Bacteriology-Mycology-II Study Section and served as its chair for three years. She serves on the editorial boards of several prestigious scientific journals and has authored over 275 articles and book chapters. She has been intimately involved in the establishment of science policy and legislation related to biomedical research and public health. Dr. Cassell has received several national and international awards and an honorary degree for her research on infectious diseases.

GARY CHRISTOPHERSON is senior advisor for force health protection at the U.S. Department of Defense, Reserve Affairs. Previously, as principal deputy assistant secretary of defense for health affairs, he managed policy, the Defense Health Program budget, and performance for the Military Health System, including the $16 billion TRICARE health care system and force health protection. In that role he also launched the Department of State's infectious disease surveillance and response system and served as cochair on the White House's infectious disease surveillance and response subcommittee. He has also been a key figure in the department's force health protection initiative against anthrax. In early 1998 he also served as the acting assistant secretary of defense for health affairs. Joining the Department of Defense in 1994, he has served as health affairs acting principal deputy assistant secretary and senior advisor where he provided advice on a wide range of health issues and managed the relationships with the White House and other federal agencies. Previously, he served 2 years (1992–1994) with the Office of Presidential Personnel at the White House and the Presidential Transition Office. As associate director, he managed the President's appointments to the Departments of Health and Human Services and Defense as well as 10 other departments. Prior to that, he served in a number of senior health positions with the Congress and with public and private health agencies.

GORDON DEFRIESE, Ph.D., is professor of social medicine and professor of medicine (in the Division of General Medicine and Clinical Epidemiology) at the University of North Carolina, Chapel Hill School of Medicine. In addition, he holds appointments as professor of epidemiology and health policy and administration in the UNC-CH School of Public Health and as professor of dental ecology in the UNC-CH School of Dentistry. From 1986–2000, he served as co-director of the Robert Wood Johnson Clinical Scholars Program, co-sponsored by the UNC-CH School of Medicine and the Cecil G. Sheps Center for Health Services Research. He received his Ph.D. from the University of Kentucky College of Medicine. Some of his research interests are in the areas of health promotion and disease prevention, medical sociology, primary health care, rural health care, cost–benefit analyses, and cost effectiveness. He is a past president of the Association for Health Services Research and a fellow of the New York Academy of Medicine. He is founder of the Partnership for Prevention, a coalition of private-sector business and industry organizations, voluntary health organizations, and state and federal public health agencies based in Washington, D.C. that have joined together to work toward the elevation of disease prevention among the nation's health policy priorities. He is an at-large member of the National Board of Medical Examiners. Since 1994 he has served as President and CEO of the North Carolina Institute of Medicine. He is Editor-in-Chief and Publisher of the North Carolina Medical Journal.

CEDRIC E. DUMONT, M.D., is medical director for the Office of Medical Services (MED) at the U.S. Department of State. Dr. Dumont graduated from Columbia University with a B.A. in 1975 and obtained his medical degree from Tufts University School of Medicine in 1980. Dr. Dumont is a board-certified internist with subspecialty training in infectious diseases. He completed his internal medicine residency in 1983 and infectious diseases fellowship in 1988 at Georgetown University Hospital in Washington, D.C. Dr. Dumont has been a medical practitioner for over 19 years, 2 of which included service in the Peace Corps. Since joining the Department of State in 1990, he has had substantial experience overseas in Dakar, Bamako, Kinshasa, and Brazzaville. For the past 3 years, as the medical director for the Department of State, Dr. Dumont has promoted the health of all U.S. government employees serving overseas by encouraging their participation in a comprehensive health maintenance program and by facilitating their access to high-quality medical care. Dr. Dumont is a very strong supporter of the professional development and advancement of MED's highly qualified professional staff. In addition, he has supported and encouraged the use of an electronic medical record, which will be able to monitor the health of all its beneficiaries, not only during a specific assignment but also throughout their careers in the Foreign Service.

JESSE L. GOODMAN, M.D., M.P.H., was professor of medicine and chief of infectious diseases at the University of Minnesota and is now serving as deputy director for the Food and Drug Administration's (FDA) Center for Biologics Evaluation and Research, where he is active in a broad range of scientific, public health, and policy issues. After joining the FDA commissioner's office, he has worked closely with several centers and helped coordinate FDA's response to the antimicrobial resistance problem. He was cochair of a recently formed federal interagency task force which developed the national Public Health Action Plan on antimicrobial resistance. He graduated from Harvard College and attended the Albert Einstein College of Medicine followed by training in internal medicine, hematology, oncology, and infectious diseases at the University of Pennsylvania and University of California, Los Angeles, where he was also chief medical resident. He received his master's of public health from the University of Minnesota. He has been active in community public health activities, including creating an environmental health partnership in St. Paul, Minnesota. In recent years, his laboratory's research has focused on the molecular pathogenesis of tickborne diseases. His laboratory isolated the etiological intracellular agent of the emerging tickborne infection, human granulocytic ehrlichiosis, and identified its leukocyte receptor. He has also been an active clinician and teacher and has directed or participated in major multicenter clinical studies. He is a fellow of the Infectious Diseases Society of America and, among several honors, has been elected to the American Society for Clinical Investigation.

RENU GUPTA, M.D., is vice president and head of U.S. Clinical Research and Development at Novartis Pharmaceuticals. Previously, she was vice president of medical, safety, and therapeutics at Covance. Dr. Gupta is a board certified pediatrician, with subspeciality training in infectious diseases from Children's Hospital of Philadelphia, and the University of Pennsylvania. She was also a postdoctoral research fellow in microbiology at the University of Pennsylvania and the Wistar Institute of Anatomy and Biology, where she conducted research on the pathogenesis of infectious diseases. Dr. Gupta received her M.B.,Ch.B with distinction from the University of Zambia, where she examined the problem of poor compliance in the treatment of tuberculosis in rural and urban Africa. She is currently active in a number of professional societies, including the Infectious Diseases Society of America and the American Society of Microbiology. She is a frequent presenter at the Interscience Conference on Antimicrobial Agents and Chemotherapy and other major congresses and has been published in leading infectious diseases periodicals. From 1989 to mid-1998, Dr. Gupta was with Bristol-Myers Squibb Company, where she directed clinical research as well as strategic planning for the Infectious Diseases and Immunology Divisions. For the past several years, her work has focused on a better understanding of the problem of emerging infections. This has led to her pioneering efforts in establishing the Global Antimicrobial Surveillance Program, SENTRY, a private-academic-public sector partnership. Dr. Gupta chaired the steering committee for the SENTRY Antimicrobial Surveillance Program. She remains active in women and children's health issues, and is currently furthering education and outreach initiatives. More recently Dr. Gupta has been instrumental in the formation of the Harvard-Pharma Management Board, of which she is a member, to further the educational goals of the Scholars in Clinical Science Program at the Harvard Medical School.

MARGARET A. HAMBURG, M.D., is vice president for biological programs, Nuclear Threat Initiative, Washington, D.C. The NTI is a new organization whose mission is to strengthen global security by reducing the risk of use of nuclear and other weapons of mass destruction and preventing their spread. Dr. Hamburg is in charge of the biological program area. Before taking on her current position, she was assistant secretary for planning and evaluation at the U.S. Department of Health and Human Services, serving as a principal policy adviser to the Secretary of Health and Human Services with responsibilities including policy formulation and analysis, the development and review of regulations and/or legislation, budget analysis, strategic planning, and the conduct and coordination of policy research and program evaluation. Prior to this, she served for almost 6 years as the commissioner of health for New York City. As chief health officer in the nation's largest city, Dr. Hamburg's many accomplishments included the design and implementation of an internationally recognized tuberculosis control program that produced dramatic declines in tuberculosis cases, the development of initiatives that raised childhood immunization rates to record levels, and the creation of the first public health bioterrorism preparedness program in the nation. She completed her internship and residency in internal medicine at the New York Hospital/Cornell University Medical Center and is certified by the American Board of Internal Medicine. Dr. Hamburg is a graduate of Harvard College and Harvard Medical School. She currently serves on the Harvard University Board of Overseers. She has been elected to membership in the Institute of Medicine, the New York Academy of Medicine, and the Council on Foreign Relations and is a fellow of the American Association for the Advancement of Science.

CAROLE A. HEILMAN, Ph.D., is director of the Division of Microbiology and Infectious Diseases (DMID) of the National Institute of Allergy and Infectious Diseases (NIAID). Dr. Heilman received her bachelor's degree in biology from Boston University in 1972 and earned her master's degree and doctorate in microbiology from Rutgers University in 1976 and

1979. Dr. Heilman began her career at the National Institutes of Health as a postdoctoral research associate with the National Cancer Institute, where she carried out research on the regulation of gene expression during cancer development. In 1986 she came to NIAID as the influenza and viral respiratory diseases program officer in DMID, and in 1988 she was appointed chief of the respiratory diseases branch, where she coordinated the development of acellular pertussis vaccines. She joined the Division of AIDS as deputy director in 1997 and was responsible for developing the Innovation Grant Program for approaches in HIV vaccine research. She is the recipient of several notable awards for outstanding achievement. Throughout her extramural career Dr. Heilman has contributed articles on vaccine design and development to many scientific journals and has served as a consultant to the World Bank and the World Health Organization. She is also a member of several professional societies, including the Infectious Diseases Society of America, the American Society for Microbiology, and the American Society of Virology.

JAMES M. HUGHES, M.D., received his B.A. in 1966 and M.D. in 1971 from Stanford University. He completed a residency in internal medicine at the University of Washington and a fellowship in infectious diseases at the University of Virginia. He is board-certified in internal medicine, infectious diseases, and preventive medicine. He first joined the Centers for Disease Control and Prevention as an epidemic intelligence service officer in 1973. During his CDC career, he has worked primarily in the areas of foodborne disease and infection control in health care settings. He became director of the National Center for Infectious Diseases in 1992. The center is currently working to address domestic and global challenges posed by emerging infectious diseases and the threat of bioterrorism. He is a fellow of the American College of Physicians, the Infectious Diseases Society of America, and the American Association for the Advancement of Science. He is an assistant surgeon general in the U.S. Public Health Service.

SAMUEL L. KATZ, M.D., is Wilburt C. Davison professor and chairman emeritus of pediatrics at Duke University Medical Center. He has concentrated his research on infectious diseases, focusing primarily on vaccine research, development and policy. Dr. Katz has served on a number of scientific advisory committees and is the recipient of many prestigious awards and honorary fellowships in international organizations. He earned his M.D. at Harvard Medical School and completed his residency training at Boston hospitals. He became a staff member at Children's Hospital, working with Nobel laureate John Enders, during which time they developed the attenuated measles virus vaccine now used throughout the world. He has chaired the Committee on Infectious Diseases of the American Academy of Pediatrics (the Redbook Committee), the Advisory Committee on Immunization Practices (ACIP) of the Centers for Disease Control and

Prevention, the Vaccine Priorities Study of the Institute of Medicine (IOM), and several World Health Organization (WHO) and Children's Vaccine Initiative panels on vaccines. He is a member of many scientific advisory committees including those of the NIH, IOM, and WHO. Dr. Katz's published studies include abundant original scientific articles, chapters in textbooks, and many abstracts, editorials, and reviews. He is the coeditor of a textbook on pediatric infectious diseases and has given many named lectures in the United States and abroad. Currently he co-chairs the Indo-US Vaccine Action Program as well as the National Network for Immunization Information (NNII).

COLONEL PATRICK KELLEY, M.D., M.P.H., Dr.P.H., is Director of the Department of Defense Global Emerging Infections System and the Director of the Division of Preventive Medicine at the Walter Reed Army Institute of Research (WRAIR), Silver Spring, Maryland. He obtained his M.D. from the University of Virginia and a Dr.P.H. in infectious disease epidemiology from the Johns Hopkins Bloomberg School of Public Health. He is board-certified in general preventive medicine and a fellow of the American College of Preventive Medicine. For many years he directed the Army General Preventive Medicine Residency at WRAIR. Colonel Kelley has extensive experience leading military infectious disease studies and in managing domestic and international public health surveillance efforts. He has spoken before professional audiences in over 15 countries and has authored or co-authored over 40 scientific papers and book chapters on a variety of infectious disease and preventive medicine topics. He serves as the specialty editor for a textbook entitled, Military Preventive Medicine: Mobilization and Deployment.

MARCELLE LAYTON, M.D., is the assistant commissioner for the Bureau of Communicable Diseases at the New York City Department of Health. The bureau is responsible for the surveillance and control of 51 infectious diseases and conditions reportable under the New York City Health Code. Current areas of concern include antibiotic resistance; foodborne, waterborne, and tickborne diseases; hepatitis C; and biological disaster planning for the potential threats of bioterrorism and pandemic influenza. Dr. Layton received her medical degree from Duke University. She completed an internal medicine residency at the University Health Science Center in Syracuse, New York, and an infectious disease fellowship at Yale University. In addition, Dr. Layton spent two years with the Centers for Disease Control and Prevention as a fellow in the Epidemic Intelligence Service, where she was assigned to the New York City Department of Health. In the past, she has volunteered or worked with the Indian Health Service, the Alaskan Native Health Service, and clinics in northwestern Thailand and central Nepal.

CARLOS LOPEZ, Ph.D., is a research fellow with Research Acquisitions, Eli Lilly Research Laboratories. He received his Ph.D. from the University of Minnesota in 1970. Dr. Lopez was awarded the NTRDA postdoctoral fellowship. After his fellowship he was appointed assistant professor of pathology at the University of Minnesota, where he did his research on cytomegalovirus infections in renal transplant recipients and the consequences of those infections. He was next appointed assistant member and head of the Laboratory of Herpesvirus Infections at the Sloan Kettering Institute for Cancer Research, where his research focused on herpes virus infections and the resistance mechanisms involved. Dr. Lopez's laboratory contributed to the immunological analysis of the earliest AIDS patients at the beginning of the AIDS epidemic in New York. He is coauthor of one of the seminal publications on this disease as well as many scientific papers and is coeditor of six books. Dr. Lopez has been a consultant to numerous agencies and organizations, including the National Institutes of Health, the Department of Veterans Affairs, and the American Cancer Society.

LYNN MARKS, M.D., is board certified in internal medicine and infectious diseases. He was on faculty at the University of South Alabama College of Medicine in the Infectious Diseases department focusing on patient care, teaching and research. His academic research interest was on the molecular genetics of bacterial pathogenicity. He subsequently joined SmithKline Beecham's (now GlaxoSmithKline) anti-infectives clinical group and later progressed to global head of the Consumer Healthcare division Medical and Regulatory group. He then returned to pharmaceutical research and development as global head of the Infectious Diseases Therapeutic Area Strategy Team for GlaxoSmithKline.

STEPHEN S. MORSE, Ph.D., is director of the Center for Public Health Preparedness at the Mailman School of Public Health of Columbia University, and a faculty member in the Epidemiology Department. Dr. Morse recently returned to Columbia from 4 years in government service as program manager at the Defense Advanced Research Projects Agency (DARPA), where he co-directed the Pathogen Countermeasures program and subsequently directed the Advanced Diagnostics program. Before coming to Columbia, he was assistant professor of virology at The Rockefeller University in New York, where he remains an adjunct faculty member. Dr. Morse is the editor of two books, *Emerging Viruses* (Oxford University Press, 1993; paperback, 1996) (selected by "American Scientist" for its list of "100 Top Science Books of the 20th Century"), and *The Evolutionary Biology of Viruses* (Raven Press, 1994). He currently serves as a Section Editor of the CDC journal "Emerging Infectious Diseases" and was formerly an Editor-in-Chief of the Pasteur Institute's journal "Research in Virology". Dr. Morse was chair and principal organizer of the 1989 NIAID/NIH Conference on Emerging Viruses (for which he originated the term and concept of emerging viruses/infections); served as a member of the

Institute of Medicine-National Academy of Sciences' Committee on Emerging Microbial Threats to Health (and chaired its Task Force on Viruses), and was a contributor to its report, *Emerging Infections* (1992); was a member of the IOM's Committee on Xenograft Transplantation; currently serves on the Steering Committee of the Institute of Medicine's Forum on Emerging Infections, and has served as an adviser to WHO (World Health Organization), PAHO (Pan-American Health Organization), FDA, the Defense Threat Reduction Agency (DTRA), and other agencies. He is a fellow of the New York Academy of Sciences and a past chair of its Microbiology Section. He was the founding chair of ProMED (the nonprofit international Program to Monitor Emerging Diseases) and was one of the originators of ProMED-mail, an international network inaugurated by ProMED in 1994 for outbreak reporting and disease monitoring using the Internet. Dr. Morse received his Ph.D. from the University of Wisconsin-Madison.

MICHAEL T. OSTERHOLM, Ph.D., M.P.H., is director of the Center for Infectious Disease Research and Policy at the University of Minnesota where he is also professor at the School of Public Health. Previously, Dr. Osterholm was the state epidemiologist and chief of the Acute Disease Epidemiology Section for the Minnesota Department of Health. He has received numerous research awards from the National Institute of Allergy and Infectious Diseases and the Centers for Disease Control and Prevention (CDC). He served as principal investigator for the CDC-sponsored Emerging Infections Program in Minnesota. He has published more than 240 articles and abstracts on various emerging infectious disease problems and is the author of the best selling book, Living Terrors: What America Needs to Know to Survive the Coming Bioterrorist Catastrophe. He is past president of the Council of State and Territorial Epidemiologists. He currently serves on the National Academy of Sciences, Institute of Medicine (IOM) Forum on Emerging Infections. He has also served on the IOM Committee, Food Safety, Production to Consumption, the IOM Committee on the Department of Defense Persian Gulf Syndrome Comprehensive Clinical Evaluation Program and as a reviewer for the IOM report on chemical and biological terrorism.

GARY A. ROSELLE, M.D., received his M.D. from Ohio State University School of Medicine in 1973. He served his residency at Northwestern University School of Medicine and his Infectious Diseases fellowship at the University of Cincinnati School of Medicine. Dr. Roselle is the Program Director for Infectious Diseases for VA Central Office in Washington, D.C., as well as the Chief of the Medical Service at the Cincinnati VA Medical Center. He is a professor of medicine in the Department of Internal Medicine, Division of Infectious Diseases at the University of Cincinnati College of Medicine. Dr. Roselle serves on several national advisory committees. In addition, he is currently heading the Emerging Pathogens Initiative for the

Department of Veterans Affairs. Dr. Roselle has received commendations from the Cincinnati Medical Center Director, the Under Secretary for Health for the Department of Veterans Affairs, and the Secretary of Veterans Affairs for his work in the infectious diseases program for the Department of Veterans Affairs. He has been an invited speaker at several national and international meetings, and has published over 80 papers and several book chapters.

DAVID M. SHLAES, M.D., Ph.D., is Vice President and Therapeutic Area Co-Leader for Infectious Diseases at Wyeth. Before joining Wyeth, Dr. Shlaes was professor of medicine at the Case Western Reserve University School of Medicine and chief of the Infectious Diseases Section and the Clinical Microbiology Unit at the Veterans Affairs Medical Center in Cleveland, Ohio. His major research interest has been the mechanisms and epidemiology of antimicrobial resistance in bacteria where he has published widely. He has recently become more involved in the area of public policy as it relates to the discovery and development of antibiotics. He has served on the Institute of Medicine's Forum on Emerging Infections since 1996.

JANET SHOEMAKER is director of the American Society for Microbiology's (ASM) Public Affairs Office, a position she has held since 1989. She is responsible for managing the legislative and regulatory affairs of this 42,000-member organization, the largest single biological science society in the world. She has served as principal investigator for a project funded by the National Science Foundation (NSF) to collect and disseminate data on the job market for recent doctorates in microbiology and has played a key role in ASM projects, including production of the ASM *Employment Outlook in the Microbiological Sciences* and *The Impact of Managed Care and Health System Change on Clinical Microbiology*. Previously, she held positions as assistant director of public affairs for ASM; as ASM coordinator of the U.S./U.S.S.R. Exchange Program in Microbiology, a program sponsored and coordinated by the National Science Foundation and the U.S. Department of State; and as a freelance editor and writer. She received her baccalaureate, cum laude, from the University of Massachusetts and is a graduate of George Washington University's programs in public policy and editing and publications. She has served as commissioner to the Commission on Professionals in Science and Technology and as the ASM representative to the ad hoc Group for Medical Research Funding and is a member of Women in Government Relations, the American Society of Association Executives, and the American Association for the Advancement of Science. She has coauthored published articles on research funding, biotechnology, biological weapons control, and public policy issues related to microbiology.

P. FREDERICK SPARLING, M.D., is J. Herbert Bate professor emeritus of medicine, microbiology and immunology at the University of North

Carolina (UNC) at Chapel Hill and is director of the North Carolina Sexually Transmitted Infections Research Center. Previously, he served as chair of the Department of Medicine and chair of the Department of Microbiology and Immunology at UNC. He was president of the Infectious Disease Society of America in 1996–1997. He was also a member of the Institute of Medicine's Committee on Microbial Threats to Health (1991–1992). Dr. Sparling's laboratory research is in the molecular biology of bacterial outer-membrane proteins involved in pathogenesis, with a major emphasis on gonococci and meningococci. His current studies focus on the biochemistry and genetics of iron-scavenging mechanisms used by gonococci and meningococci and the structure and function of the gonococcal porin proteins. He is pursuing the goal of a vaccine for gonorrhea.

KAYE WACHSMUTH, Ph.D., serves as deputy administrator of the Office of Public Health and Science in the USDA's Food Safety and Inspection Service. Before joining the USDA, she was the deputy director for programs at the Food and Drug Administration's Center for Food Safety and Applied Nutrition. Dr. Wachsmuth was with the Centers for Disease Control and Prevention in Atlanta from 1972 to 1994, where she was deputy director of the Division of Bacterial and Mycotic Diseases from 1991 to 1994, and chief of the Enteric Diseases Laboratory Section from 1985 to 1991. While at CDC she developed programs and conducted studies in the areas of molecular epidemiology and bacterial pathogenesis. She also worked extensively in Southeast Asia and South America to establish laboratory-based diarrheal disease surveillance programs. In addition to her positions at the FDA and CDC, Dr. Wachsmuth chairs the National Advisory Committee on Microbiological Criteria for Foods and the Codex Committee for Food Hygiene and is a member of the World Health Organization's (WHO) Expert Advisory Panel on Food Safety. Dr. Wachsmuth received her B.S. from Stetson University, Deland, Florida, and her Ph.D. in microbiology from the University of Tennessee. She is a fellow of the Infectious Diseases Society of America and the American Academy of Microbiology. She has received awards for benchmark epidemiological investigations of Legionnaire's disease, cholera in Latin America, drug-resistant tuberculosis, hantavirus in the western United States, and diphtheria in the former Soviet Union. The author of more than 160 scientific papers, she is on the editorial board of scientific journals and is editor of a book on cholera.

C. DOUGLAS WEBB, Jr., Ph.D., received his bachelor's degree in biology from Emory University and his master's and doctoral degrees in microbiology from the University of Georgia. He served in the Public Health Service at the Centers for Disease Control and Prevention (CDC) as both a research microbiologist and supervisory microbiologist. After the CDC, Dr. Webb went to Pfizer Pharmaceuticals and was involved in the development of ampicillin-sulbactam, carbenicillin, cefoperazone, fluconazole, azithromycin, and trovafloxacin. Dr. Webb is Senior Medical Director in Infectious Diseases in U.S. Medicines at Bristol-Myers Squibb, working on the strategy and development for the antiinfective portfolio.

SPEAKERS

ROY M. ANDERSON, Ph.D., F.R.S., has recently moved with his research group to head a new Department of Infectious Disease Epidemiology in the Medical School at Imperial College, University of London. He was previously Linacre Professor at the University of Oxford and founding Director of the Wellcome Trust Centre for the Epidemiology of Infectious Disease at the University of Oxford. His research interests center on the epidemiology, evolution, and control of infectious diseases using multidisciplinary approaches to further understanding. He has worked and published widely on a wide range of infectious disease agents, including HIV, the malarial parasite, the prion etiological agents of spongiform encephalopathies, helminth parasites, childhood vaccine preventable viral and bacterial infections, dengue virus, antibiotic resistant bacteria, and the pneumococcal bacteria. He is a fellow of the Royal Society in the United Kingdom and a foreign member of the Institute of Medicine.

KENNETH D. BLOEM, M.P.H., has served in leadership positions at Georgetown University Medical Center (as CEO), Stanford University Hospital (as CEO), University of Chicago Hospital and Clinics (as COO/EVP), and Boston University (as Associate Vice President of Health Affairs). In the corporate health sector, Mr. Bloem was CEO of the Advisory Board Company, a for-profit strategy and research membership company. He was a board member of Allegiance, Inc., a $4.5 billion health products and distribution company from its founding to its acquisition by Cardinal, Inc. He currently sits on the boards of a number of medium and early stage health companies. Earlier in his career, Mr. Bloem served as public health officer/epidemiologist with the World Health Organization's successful smallpox eradication program in Bangladesh and in Central Africa. He was a Peace Corps volunteer in Malaysia and in Zaire from 1968 to 1972. Mr. Bloem has a master's degree in health policy and management from the Harvard School of Public Health. He has been a visiting lecturer at Harvard, at the University of Chicago, at Stanford University School of Medicine and at Georgetown University's Graduate School of Business. He served on the editorial board of *Inquiry*, on two advisory committees to the Robert Wood Johnson Foundation, on the Institute of Medicine's Committee on Implementing the Graduate Medical Education Trust Fund, and on the Executive Committee of the University Health System Consortium. He also served on the founding Board of Directors of the Howard University Hospital. Mr.

Bloem is a Senior Fellow at the Johns Hopkins Center for Civilian Biodefense Strategies as well as Adjunct Associate Professor of International Health at Boston University School of Public Health. He is active as a consultant and speaker on the topics of bioterrorism, the relationship between public health and medical delivery, and on future trends in U.S. health care.

DONALD S. BURKE, M.D., is professor of international health and epidemiology and Director of the Center for Immunization Research at the Johns Hopkins Bloomberg School of Public Health. Previously, he served 23 years at the Walter Reed Army Institute of Research, including six years at the Armed Forces Research Institute of Medical Sciences in Bangkok. His research focuses on the epidemiology and prevention of human epidemic virus diseases including HIV/AIDS, dengue, flavivirus encephalitis, and hepatitis. He is past president of the American Society of Tropical Medicine. He has served on the NRC Roundtable for the Development of Drugs and Vaccines Against AIDS, and the NRC Committee on Climate, Ecology, Infectious Diseases, and Human Health (as chairman), and is currently a member of the IOM Committee to Review the Department of Defense Global Emerging Infections Surveillance and Response System and the IOM Committee on Emerging Microbial Threats to Health in the 21st Century.

STEPHEN L. COCHI, M.D., M.P.H., is director of the Global Immunization Division and associate director for Global Immunization in the National Immunization Program at the Centers for Disease Control and Prevention (CDC). He holds a B.S. from the Massachusetts Institute of Technology, an M.D. from Duke University, and an M.P.H. from Emory University, and completed residency training in pediatrics at the Massachusetts General Hospital and in preventive medicine at the CDC. Dr. Cochi is board certified by the American Board of Pediatrics and the American Board of Preventive Medicine. Dr. Cochi has spent 22 years at CDC working in the field of immunization. He currently leads CDC's global immunization activities and directs a $130 million per year annual program with 90 CDC staff providing technical and programmatic support, as well as vaccine grants (through UNICEF), as a major partner in the global polio eradication initiative, global measles control and mortality reduction initiative, and other priority global immunization activities under the umbrella of the Global Alliance for Vaccines and Immunization. His division works closely with U.N. agencies and private sector partners, including WHO, UNICEF, Pan American Health Organization, Rotary International, the United Nations Foundation, American Red Cross, International Federation of Red Cross and Red Crescent Societies, the World Bank, and Ministries of Health in developing and middle income countries. Dr. Cochi has authored or co-authored approximately 100 scientific journal articles and book chapters on vaccines and vaccine-preventable diseases, and more than 130 CDC publications including MMWR articles. He has served frequently as an expert consultant and lecturer on international immunization issues for WHO and other international organizations. He is a Fellow of the American Academy of Pediatrics and the Infectious Diseases Society of America, and a member of the American Public Health Association, Pediatric Infectious Diseases Society, and American Epidemiological Society.

JEFFREY I. COHEN, M.D., is head of the Medical Virology Section of the Laboratory of Clinical Investigation at the National Institutes of Health (NIH). He graduated from Johns Hopkins University Medical School and was an intern and resident at Duke University Medical Center. After a research fellowship at NIH where he contributed to the development of the inactivated hepatitis A virus vaccine, he received training in infectious diseases at Harvard Medical School. His laboratory at NIH studies molecular genetics and pathogenesis of viral infections, particularly the human herpesvirus family. He attends on the infectious disease service and is a principal investigator on clinical virology studies. He is a member of the American Society for Clinical Investigation and a fellow of the Infectious Diseases Society of America.

SUSANNA CUNNINGHAM-RUNDLES, Ph.D., is professor of immunology and Vice Chairman for Academic Affairs in the Department of Pediatrics of Cornell University Weill Medical College in New York City. She is Associate Program Director of the National Institutes of Health Children's Clinical Research Center at Cornell and directs the Immunology Research Laboratory. Dr. Cunningham-Rundles has served as a study section member and as chair of the NIH Microbial Immunology Review Group Study Section, AIDS and Related Diseases, ARR-1. She chaired the Scientific Advisory Panel, National Institute of Child Health and Human Development: Adolescent Medicine HIV/AIDS Research Network. Dr. Cunningham-Rundles is a member of the Grant Review Committee of the Pediatric AIDS Foundation and of the Scientific Advisory Committee for the American Foundation for AIDS Research. She is a fellow of the American Academy of Microbiology, the American Academy of Nutrition, served on the Board of Governors of the New York Academy of Sciences, and chaired the Conference Committee. She was the 1993 recipient of the Key To Life Award of The Children's Blood Foundation and was awarded the DeWitt Clinton Award in 1999. Dr. Cunningham-Rundles received her Ph.D. in Biochemical Genetics from New York University and was a postdoctoral fellow in immunobiology and immunogenetics at Sloan Kettering Institute of the Memorial Sloan Kettering Cancer Center. She was appointed subsequently as head of the Cellular Immunology Laboratory and became Assistant Director of the blood bank. Dr. Cunningham Rundles joined the faculty of the Cornell University Weill Medical Center in 1986. She was the first to define the cellular immune defect of AIDS and has continued to make contributions to this field. The theme of Dr. Cunningham-Rundles' research is the development of the immune system in response to encounter with microbes. She is interested in global health issues, especially during the perinatal period and was a U.S. delegate to the Indo-U.S. Workshop on Nutrition of Women, Infants, and Children, Hyderabad, India, February 2000. In addition to more than 100 publications in scientific journals, Dr. Cunningham-Rundles has edited two books "Nutrient Modulation of Immune Response" (Marcel Dekker, Inc., 1993) and "Persistent Bacterial Infections" (American Society of Microbiology, 2000).

RAYMOND H. CYPESS, D.V.M., Ph.D., is President and CEO of American Type Culture Collection (ATCC), Manassas, Virginia and Principal Investigator for ATCC's Malaria Research and Reference Reagent Resource Center (MR4) contract. Dr. Cypess was an associate professor of epidemiology and microbiology at the University of Pittsburgh School of Public Health from 1970 to 1973, professor and chairman at the New York State College of Veterinary Medicine from 1977 to 1987, and dean of the College of Graduate Health Sciences as well as professor of microbiology, immunology and comparative medicine, and Vice Provost for Research and Research Training at the University of Tennessee, Memphis from 1988 to 1993. Dr. Cypess is a member of the Board of Directors of Commonwealth Biotechnologies, Inc., a biotechnology company, and Mid Atlantic Medical, an HMO. Dr. Cypess is a fellow of the Infectious Diseases Society of America and a member of the American Epidemiology Society. Dr. Cypess received a B.S. in biology from Brooklyn College, a B. Agri. from the University of Illinois, a D.V.M. from the University of Illinois, and a Ph.D. in parasitology from the University of North Carolina.

CIRO A. DE QUADROS, M.D., M.P.H., completed his medical studies in Brazil and received his M.P.H. from the National School of Public Health in Rio de Janeiro. He was involved with pioneering experiences for the development of strategies of surveillance and containment for smallpox eradication and in 1970 joined the World Health Organization (WHO) as Chief Epidemiologist for the Smallpox Eradication Program in Ethiopia. He transferred to the Pan American Health Organization (PAHO) in 1997 to serve as the Senior Advisor on Immunizations. He directed the successful efforts of polio eradication from the Western Hemisphere and at present is the Director of the Division of Vaccines and Immunization at PAHO. Dr. de Quadros was a member of the IOM Committees "Microbial Threats to Health in the United States" and "Children's Vaccine Initiative: Planning Alternatives Strategies Toward Full U.S. Participation". He is also an Associate Adjunct Professor at the Johns Hopkins School of Hygiene and Public Health, and an Associate Professor at the School of Medicine of Case Western Reserve University. He has participated in and presented papers at over 100 conferences throughout the world and has received several international awards including the 1993 Prince Mahidol Award and the 2000 Albert B. Sabin Gold Medal.

WALTER R. DOWDLE, Ph.D., is a member of The Task Force for Child Survival and Development, Atlanta, Georgia where he serves as Director of the Malarone Donation Program and a consultant to the World Health Organization (WHO) on the Global Poliomyelitis Eradication Initiative. Prior to joining The Task Force, Dr. Dowdle was Deputy Director for the Centers for Disease Control and Prevention (CDC). He was Director of the WHO Collaborating Center for Influenza from 1968–1979 and a continuous consultant to WHO for virus diseases. He was Associate Professor, School of Public Health, University of North Carolina, 1964–1984 and Honorary Fellow, John Curtin School for Medical Research, The Australian National University, Canberra, 1972–1973. During his CDC career, Dr. Dowdle served as CDC Associate Director for HIV/AIDS; Director, Center for Infectious Diseases; CDC Assistant Director for Science; Director, Virology Division; Chief, Respiratory Virology Unit; and a participant in other disease prevention assignments. Dr. Dowdle has had extensive experience in virus research, vaccine development/evaluation, and formulation of immunization policy. His current active scientific interests include polio, influenza, HIV, and malaria.

DIANE E. GRIFFIN, M.D., Ph.D., is professor and chair of the Department of Molecular Microbiology and Immunology at the Johns Hopkins School of Public Health with joint appointments in Medicine and Neurology in the School of Medicine. She graduated from Stanford University School of Medicine with a M.D. and a Ph.D. in immunology. She was an intern and resident at Stanford and an infectious diseases and virology fellow at the Johns Hopkins School of Medicine. She is a member of the Vaccine and Related Products Advisory Panel for the FDA, the Board of Scientific Councilors at the NINDS, the Step 1 Committee for the U.S. Medical Licensing Examination, Research Advisory Committee for the National Multiple Sclerosis Society and the Research Advisory Committee for the Alberta Heritage Foundation for Medical Research. She is past president of the American Society for Virology and past member of the Steering Committee on Respiratory Virus Infections of the WHO. Her laboratory at Johns Hopkins studies the pathogenesis of viral infections, particularly alphavirus encephalitis and the effect of measles on immune responses. She is the recent recipient of a grant from the Gates Foundation to develop a measles vaccine that can be used in young infants. She is a member of the American Society for Clinical Investigation, the American Neurological Association and a fellow of the Infectious Diseases Society of America and the American Association for the Advancement of Science. She has published more than 200 articles in the scientific literature.

BEATRICE H. HAHN, M.D., is professor of medicine and microbiology at the University at Alabama at Birmingham. She received her medical degree summa cum laude from the University of Munich in Germany where she subsequently interned at the Department of Internal Medicine. She did her postdoctoral training in the Laboratory of Tumor Cell Biology at the National Cancer Institute. Her current research activities are centered on studies of the origins and evolution of primate lentiviruses. In particular, Dr. Hahn's group is characterizing natural SIV reservoirs using a variety of different approaches including non-invasive testing of highly endangered wild primate populations. The goal of these studies is to assess current human risk of acquiring such zoonotic infections. She is a member of the National Institutes of Health AIDS Vaccine Research Committee which is chaired by Dr. David Baltimore and a member of the Board of Scientific Counselors–Subcommittee B at the National Cancer Institute. She has authored or co-authored over 100 papers and is editor of AIDS Research and Human Retroviruses.

DONALD A. HENDERSON, M.D., currently is director of the newly created Office of Public Health Preparedness, which coordinates national response to public health emergencies. Dr. Henderson directed the World Health Organization's global smallpox eradication campaign and was instrumental in 1974 in initiating WHO's global program of immunization, which is now vaccinating 80 percent of the world's children against six major diseases and has a goal of eradicating poliomyelitis. Dr. Henderson is a Johns Hopkins University Distinguished Service Professor with appointments in the departments of epidemiology and international health at the Bloomberg School of Public Health. For the past four years, he has directed the Johns Hopkins Center for Civilian Biodefense Studies, of which he is a founding director. The center was established to increase awareness of the medical and public health threats posed by biological weapons. From 1977 through August 1990, Dr. Henderson was dean of the Johns Hopkins School of Public Health. He rejoined the Hopkins faculty in June 1995 after five years of federal government service in which he served initially as Associate Director, Office of Science and Technology Policy, Executive Office of the President and later as Deputy Assistant Secretary and Senior Science Advisor in the Department of Health and Human Services. Dr. Henderson has been recognized for his work by many institutions and governments. In 1986, he received the National Medal of Science, presented by the President of the United States. He is the recipient of the National Academy of Sciences' highest award, the Public Welfare Medal, and, with two colleagues, he shared the Japan Prize. Most recently he received from the Royal Society of Medicine the Edward Jenner Medal. In all, 13 universities have conferred honorary degrees and 14 countries have honored him with awards and decorations.

ROBERT P. KADLEC, M.D., M.T.M.H., is a physician and colonel in the U.S. Air Force. He presently serves as a Professor of Military Strategy and Operations at the National War College at Fort McNair, DC. A Distinguished Graduate of the U.S. Air Force Academy, he earned his M.D. from the Uniformed Services University of the Health Sciences (USUHS). He holds a master's degree in tropical medicine and hygiene from USUHS and completed his residency in General Preventive Medicine & Public Health at Walter Reed Army Institute of Research. He also holds a master of arts degree in National Security Studies from Georgetown University. Dr. Kadlec has served as a physician for both Air Force and Joint Special Operations Commands. He also served as a Senior Assistant for Counterproliferation in the Office of the Secretary of Defense for Policy. In this capacity, he represented the Secretary of Defense on the U.S. delegation to the Biological Weapons and Toxins Convention in Geneva, Switzerland and also served as a United Nations Special Commission biological weapons inspector in Iraq. He has worked on a range of policy issues concerning the nonproliferation and counterproliferation of biological weapons. He most recently served as a special advisor for biological warfare issues to the U.S.A.F. Surgeon General. He is an assistant clinical professor of military medicine at USUHS.

MARLO LIBEL, M.D., M.P.H., is an epidemiologist in the Communicable Diseases Program, Disease Prevention and Control Division, at the Pan American Health Organization (PAHO). As regional advisor on communicable diseases in the Americas, he is responsible for the implementation of the Regional Plan for Surveillance and Control of Emerging and Reemerging Diseases and the revision of the International Health Regulations. Prior to that, he was responsible for the implementation of the Core Data/Country Profile database system which involved gathering, compiling, and validating core health data in collaboration with PAHO's country offices. Before this, he coordinated PAHO's response to the cholera epidemic; elaborated a Regional Plan for the Prevention and Control of Cholera; and managed PAHO/HQ's and interagency cholera task forces. He managed a $3.8 million IDB grant for technical cooperation on cholera surveillance and control for 25 countries. He assisted in resource mobilization for cholera control with the IDB, the European Union, Swedish International Development Agency, and the Italian Cooperation. Dr. Libel was formerly chief of the Epidemiological Control Unit, at the Rio Grande do Sul State Health Department in Brazil where he was responsible for the daily technical administration and operation of the state's communicable diseases epidemiological surveillance system and immunization program. He received his medical degree in Brazil and has a master of public health degree from the Tulane School of Public Health and Tropical Medicine.

THOMAS P. MONATH, M.D., received his undergraduate degree and M.D. from Harvard University and did postgraduate training in internal medicine at the Peter Bent Brigham Hospital, Boston. Subsequently, he was Medical Officer in the Arbovirology Unit, Centers for Disease Control and Prevention (CDC) and then was visiting scientist at the Rockefeller Foundation Virus Research Laboratory, Ibadan, Nigeria, where he conducted field research on yellow fever and other arboviruses. He led investigations on the ecology of Lassa virus in West Africa, resulting in the discovery of the rodent host responsible for disease transmission to humans. From 1973–1988 he was Director of the Division of Vector-Borne Viral Diseases, CDC and was responsible for surveillance, epidemic investigations, and research on arboviruses, bubonic plague, and other zoonotic diseases. He then became Chief, Virology Division, at the U.S. Army Medical Research Institute of Infectious Diseases, where he directed research and development efforts on antiviral drugs and vaccines against hemorrhagic fever viruses and arboviruses. In 1992, Dr. Monath became Vice President, Research & Medical Affairs, OraVax Inc. (now named Acambis Inc.), a biotechnology company engaged in the development of vaccines against infectious diseases. He initiated Acambis' vaccine R&D efforts on dengue, Japanese encephalitis, West Nile, yellow fever, *Clostridium difficile,* and *Helicobacter pylori.* In 2000, Acambis was awarded the contract for manufacture of a cell-culture based smallpox vaccine, and Dr. Monath is Technical Director of this program. He is also Adjunct Professor, Harvard School of Public Health. Dr. Monath has served as Chairman of the American Committee on Arthropod-Borne Viruses, Program Chairman and Councilor of the American Society of Tropical Medicine & Hygiene, and as a member of numerous WHO, PAHO, and U.S. government committees, including the National Vaccines Advisory Committee. He has published over 300 scientific papers and book chapters and edited 5 books.

ANN E. NORWOOD, M.D., is a colonel in the U.S. Army and currently serves as associate professor of psychiatry and Associate Chairman for the Department of Psychiatry at the Uniformed Services University of the Health Sciences (USUHS). Dr. Norwood received her A.B. in psychobiology from Vassar College and M.D. from USUHS. She completed her residency in psychiatry at Letterman Army Medical Center, San Francisco. She was the chief of psychiatry at Darnall Army Community Hospital, Ft. Hood, Texas before coming to the University in 1988. She is the recipient of the William C. Porter Award given by the Association of the Military Surgeons of the United States for outstanding contributions to military psychiatry. She holds the "A" designation for her expertise in trauma and disasters from the Army Surgeon General. She serves as the Chair of the American Psychiatric Association's Committee on Psychiatric Dimensions of Disaster. Dr. Norwood has published numerous articles and chapters on the effects of trauma and violence as well as the volume, *Emotional Aftermath of the Persian Gulf War: Veterans, Families, Communities, and Nations*. Most recently, she has focused on the use of biological and chemical agents by terrorists. Dr. Norwood co-authored an article on this topic for the *Journal of the American Medical Association (JAMA)* and has spoken on psychological aspects of weapons of mass destruction to numerous audiences including the American Medical Association, the American Psychiatric Association, and the American Academy of Neurology.

ELLYN W. OGDEN, M.P.H., is the Worldwide Polio Eradication Coordinator for the U.S. Agency for International Development (USAID) and a Senior Technical Advisor for Health and Child Survival. She is responsible for the Agency's polio eradication activities and related immunization and disease control efforts now focused in 20 countries. Ms. Ogden works closely with the "Polio Partner" organizations, including WHO, UNICEF, CDC, Rotary International, NGOs, Foundations and host country governments and coordinates 14 USAID centrally-funded projects that contribute to polio eradication in the areas of research, implementation, and communication. A graduate of the Tulane School of Public Health and Tropical Medicine, Ms. Ogden has over 15 years of international public health experience in the areas of child survival, disease prevention and control, nutrition, and health and human rights. After receiving her M.P.H., she conducted clinical epidemiologic research in cancer and heart disease and taught research methodology at Louisiana State University Medical and Nursing Schools. She became a Peace Corps volunteer in Papua New Guinea where she ran a provincial health program to control tuberculosis, leprosy, and sexually transmitted diseases. Subsequently, at USAID, she became the Project Director of an Applied Health Research project and was responsible for coordinating the design and evaluation of projects in USAID's child survival portfolio. She was then a Johns Hopkins University Health and Child Survival Fellow in USAID's Latin America Bureau where she managed programs to improve children's and women's health in Central America. Ms. Ogden is an adviser on several international health advisory panels and regularly works with developing country governments, health professionals, and non-governmental organizations to improve the health of people in their country.

C. J. PETERS, M.D., graduated from Rice University and Johns Hopkins School of Medicine before an internship and residency in internal medicine at Parkland Memorial Hospital, Southwestern Medical School in Dallas. His interest in tropical medicine and virology was sparked by 5 years at an NIAID laboratory in Panama after which he spent 3 years working in immunology at the Scripps Clinic and Research Foundation. He then was at the U.S. Army Medical Research Institute of Infectious Diseases where he held several positions ranging from research scientist, division chief, to deputy commander. Subsequently he moved to the Centers for Disease Control and Prevention as head of the Special Pathogens Branch. His career includes 30 years' experience with virology, pathogenesis, and epidemiology of hemorrhagic fever viruses. He developed animal models for Rift Valley fever (RVF) virus, discovered the sensitivity of RVF virus to ribavirin and immunomodulators, and has both developed and evaluated RVF vaccines through human testing. He has worked on several arenaviruses (including lymphocytic choriomeningitis virus, Lassa fever, Bolivian hemorrhagic fever, and Argentine hemorrhagic fever) and has been active in developing therapy and vaccines for these agents as well. His experience extends to other hemorrhagic viruses including Ebola, yellow fever, and Crimean Congo hemorrhagic fever virus. Dr. Peters has authored or coauthored 300 scientific publications, including more than 70 publications on RVF virus and more than 60 publications on arenaviruses, not including reviews or textbook chapters. He has worked as a bench scientist and has supervised groups with several scientists numbering up to 50 persons. Since 2001, Dr. Peters has been at the University of Texas Medical Branch in Galveston where he is a member of the WHO Collaborating Center for Tropical Diseases and a professor in the Department of Pathology and in the Department of Microbiology and Immunology. He has extensive experience in high containment laboratory work and is incoming Director of the Biosafety Level 4 laboratory under construction at UTMB and expected to be completed in 2002.

STANLEY A. PLOTKIN, M.D., is currently a medical and scientific consultant, Aventis Pasteur, after seven years as Medical and Scientific Director, Pasteur Merieux Connaught Vaccines, Paris. He is also emeritus professor of pediatrics at the University of Pennsylvania and emeritus professor of virology at the Wistar Institute. Over the course of his career he has served as Senior Assistant Surgeon, Epidemic Intelligence Service, USPHS, director of the Division of Infectious Diseases at Children's Hospital of Philadelphia, and as associate chairman, Department of Pediatrics, University of Pennsylvania. Dr. Plotkin has developed many vaccines, including the rubella vaccine, RA27/3 strain, now exclusively used in the United States and throughout the world. He has held editorial positions with many scholarly journals and is a member of numerous professional and scientific societies, including the American Academy for the Advancement of Science, the Society for Pediatric Research, the American Society for Microbiology, the Infectious Diseases Society of America, and the American Epidemiologic Society. Dr. Plotkin has received several professional awards including the French Legion Medal of Honor (1998); the Clinical Virology Award, Pan American Group for Rapid Viral Diagnosis (1995); the Distinguished Physician Award, Pediatric Infectious Disease Society (1993); and the Bruce Medal of the American College of Physicians.

VINCENT R. RACANIELLO, Ph.D., is Higgins Professor of Microbiology at the College of Physicians and Surgeons of Columbia University. He received an A.B. degree in biology from Cornell University. In 1980, for work carried out with Dr. Peter Palese, he received a Ph.D. in biomedical sciences from Mt. Sinai School of Medicine of the City University of New York. After postdoctoral work with Dr. David Baltimore at the Massachusetts Institute of Technology, in 1982 he joined the College of Physicians and Surgeons as assistant professor of microbiology. He is the recipient of an Irma T. Hirschl Career Scientist Award, the Searle Scholars Award, the Eli Lilly Award of the American Society for Microbiology in 1992, and an NIH Merit Award. He was a Harvey Society Lecturer in 1991, was the First Lamb Professor at Vanderbilt University and presented the Hilleman Lecture at the University of Chicago in 1993. Dr. Racaniello is an editor of the Journal of Virology. He previously served as a member of the World Health Organization Steering Committee on Hepatitis/Polio, chair of the Virology Study Section of the National Institutes of Health, and co-Chair of the Gordon Conference on Viruses and Cells. Research in his laboratory has focused on the mechanisms of poliovirus replication and pathogenesis. His research has produced the first infectious clone of an RNA virus, the discovery of the cell receptor for poliovirus, and the establishment of a mouse model for poliomyelitis. These contributions have revolutionized the study of animal RNA viruses.

FRANK P. SIMIONE, M.S., is Vice President of Safety and Regulatory Affairs, and Director of Professional Services at American Type Culture Collection (ATCC), Manassas, Virginia. He has overall responsibility for internal safety and security for biological materials, as well as for ensuring control of the release and distribution of biological materials from ATCC. This includes assuring ATCC compliance with all domestic and international regulations for release and transport, and overseeing ATCC's Export Management System. Within Professional Services Mr. Simione manages the largest International Depository Authority under the Budapest Treaty for deposits in support of patent applications, and he has overall responsibility for ATCC's biorepository management contract with CDC. He has been with ATCC for 26 years, was Director of Operations from 1988 to 1996, and has been Safety Officer since 1988. Mr. Simione received a B.A. degree in biology from Temple University in 1968 and a M.S. degree in biology from Bucknell University in 1974.

CARL E. TAYLOR, M.D., M.P.H., is the founding chair of the Department of International Health at the Johns Hopkins School of Hygiene and Public Health. He was head of that department for 23 years and is now professor emeritus of International Health. Through the mid-1980s he was UNICEF Representative in China and continued to work in various roles for UNICEF. He was founding chair of the National Council for International Health (now Global Health Council) and of the International Health Section of the American Public Health Section. He was chair of the 1995 Commission on the Impact of the Expanded Program on Immunization and the Polio Eradication Initiative on Health Systems in the Americas. His doctorates in medicine and public health are from Harvard and he is Honorary Professor in two Chinese medical universities. He has worked at field level in over 60 developing countries with a particular interest in health care reform on issues such as equity, integration of services such as infection control and nutrition and of MCH and family planning, balancing the roles of public and private providers, partnerships for community empowerment and scaling up of successful programs.

STEPHEN P. TERET, J.D., M.P.H., is professor of health policy and management and associate chair for health and public policy in the Johns Hopkins School of Public Health. He is the director of the Johns Hopkins Center for Gun Policy and Research, and director of the Johns Hopkins Center for Law and the Public's Health. Professor Teret holds joint faculty appointments in pediatrics and in emergency medicine at the Johns Hopkins School of Medicine, and is Adjunct Professor of Health Law at the Georgetown University Law Center. Professor Teret has worked as a poverty lawyer and a trial lawyer in New York. Since 1979, he has been a full-time faculty member at the Johns Hopkins School of Public Health. His work includes research, teaching, and public service in the areas of injury prevention and health law. Professor Teret's work has also focused on the understanding and prevention of violence, with an emphasis on gun policy. Professor Teret is the author of many scholarly articles and books on the subject of injury epidemiology and prevention. He is a frequent lecturer at major universities throughout the country, and has served as a consultant to the President of the United States, the Attorney General, the United States Congress, federal agencies, and state legislatures. He is the recipient of distinguished career awards from the American Public Health Association and the Association of Trial Lawyers of America.

RICHARD J. WHITLEY, M.D., is Loeb Eminent Scholar Chair in Pediatrics and professor of pediatrics, microbiology, and medicine at the University of Alabama at Birmingham. Dr. Whitley also is scientist at the Cancer Research and Training Center; Associate Director of the Center for AIDS Research; and Vice-Chairman of the Department of Pediatrics at the university. Dr. Whitley is responsible for the National Institute of Allergy and Infectious Diseases Collaborative Antiviral Study Group whose role is to perform clinical trials of antiviral therapies directed against medically important viral diseases of children and adults. His other research interest is in utilizing herpes simplex for gene therapy. Active investigations are resulting in the engineering of herpes simplex virus for gene therapy of brain and liver tumors and vaccine development. Dr. Whitley received his B.A. in chemistry from Duke University and his M.D. from the George Washington University. He subsequently completed an internship in pediatrics and a fellowship in infectious diseases/virology at the University of Alabama at Birmingham. He has published over 260 articles.